Preface

Some things are too good to let go, and Behavioral Relaxation Training (BRT) is one of them. I was fortunate to be among the first wave of students to be trained in BRT and it has served us all in good stead.

Behavioral Relaxation Training—Clinical Applications with Diverse Populations is both old and new. This edition, like the original, presents the behavior analytic conceptualization of complex behavior, including relaxation, the overall approach to teaching relaxation skills to participants, the Behavioral Relaxation Scale, and enumerates the myriad research questions that remain to be addressed. To this solid base we have added new content, including an expansion of the analysis of complex behavior and the four-modality response system (4MRS), updated citations, elaborated on the utility of values clarification, and presented motivational interviewing techniques to establish rule-governed behavior (ply and pliance) related to behavior change, generally, and relaxation, specifically. To round things out, a number of new measures have been included, such as the States of Arousal and Relaxation Scale (STAR), and a description new applications of the BRS and BRT in the areas of autism spectrum disorder, pain, movement disorders, and anxiety.

Behavioral Relaxation Training—Clinical Applications with Diverse Populations, like its predecessor, describes how to employ evidenced-based relaxation assessment and training procedures addressing a variety of disorders and behaviors across the lifespan and in diverse settings. It presents problems and assessment procedures that are directly relevant to applied behavior analysts, nurses, clinical social workers, professional counselors, and psychologists. More specifically, each chapter ends with a supplement containing BACB Task List Items.

—Duane A. Lundervold
February, 2020

Acknowledgements

This work would not have been possible without the hard work and commitment of Lacy S. Hites, Angel Dunlap, Natalie (Howie) Howard, Chris Talley and Mike Buermann. Thanks go to Christine Hobbs for pointing me in the way of mindfulness and relaxation, and to Lindsay Lettow for the assistance in the mindfulness and BRT research. Though they must go nameless, it is from the research participants at SIU-C, patients at University of Kansas School of Medicine, and Plaza Primary Care and Geriatrics that have taught me much about the clinical application and benefits of BRT. Finally, none of this would have been possible without the continued professional support of David S. Kreiner, PhD, Chair, School of Kinesiology, Nutrition, and Psychological Science at the University of Central Missouri, Mila K., and Dr. Rock. Ride on, brother!

—Duane A. Lundervold
February, 2020

This book is the culmination of work of my students and colleagues over the years while at Southern Illinois University-Carbondale and elsewhere. Many people have contributed over the years, and for that I am fortunate. I have learned much.

—Roger Poppen
February, 2020

Obviously, none of this would have been possible were it not for all of the participants whom I have served over the last 29 years. They have taught me so much about myself, but have also underscored the utility of the principle outlines in this book to improve the lives of both caregiver and participant. I am also deeply indebted to my beautiful wife Tess and our four children, Chase, Savannah, Luke, and Tyler. Tess has supported me in all of my writing endeavors and I am so truly grateful for that. My academic mentor, Dr. Roger Poppen, has also played a huge role in shaping my professional journey to allow me to see the importance of this work and how it can impact the lives of those who employ it.

—John M. Guerico
February, 2020

Behavioral Relaxation Training

Clinical Applications with Diverse Populations

Third Edition

Duane A. Lundervold
University of Central Missouri

Roger Poppen
Professor Emeritus, Southern Illinois University

John M. Guercio
Benchmark Human Services

2020
Sloan Publishing
Cornwall on Hudson, NY 12520

Library of Congress Control Number: 2020942196

Cover photo: ID 53402635 © Antonio1962.| Dreamstime.com

© 2020 by Sloan Publishing, LLC

Sloan Publishing, LLC
220 Maple Road
Cornwall-on-Hudson, NY 12520

All rights reserved. No portion of this book may be reproduced, in any form or by any means, without permission in writing from the Publisher.

Printed in the United States of America

10 9 8 7 6 5 4 3 2 1

ISBN 13: 978-1-59738-099-7
ISBN 10: 1-59738-099-7

Contents

Preface   vii
Acknowledgements   viii
About the Authors   ix
Foreword by Peter Sturmey, Ph.D.   xi

1. **Stress and Coping**   1
   Two Case Studies   1
   Stress   5
   Anxiety   8
   Anger   11
   Conclusions   12
   BACB Task List (5th edition)   15

2. **Relaxation Training: An Overview**   17
   A Brief History and Description of Training Procedures   17
   Theories of Relaxation   24
   Relaxation as a Response Class   34
   Conclusions   36
   BACB Task List (5th edition)   40

3. **Assessment of Relaxation**   42
   Function-Based Assessment and Relaxation   42
   Assessment of Training   44
   Self-Report Measures of Relaxation   45
   The Behavioral Relaxation Scale (BRS)   49

Conclusions   70
BACB Task List (5th edition)   74

4. Behavioral Relaxation Training   75
Prerequisites for Training   76
Acquisition Training Procedures   78
Proficiency Training Procedures   84
Variations of Behavioral Relaxation Training   90
Focused Breathing   95
Issues That May Interfere with BRT   100
Modifications of the BRT Protocol for Diverse Populations and Individual Needs   104
Training the Trainers   107
Conclusions   109
BACB Task List (5th edition)   112

5. Neurodevelopmental Disorders   115
Intellectual Disabilities (ID)   116
Autism Spectrum Disorder (ASD)   125
Schizophrenic Spectrum Disorder (SSD)   127
Attention Deficit/Hyperactivity Disorder (ADHD)   130
Emotional Disturbance (ED)   138
Conclusions   139
BACB Task List (5th edition)   147

6. Pain, Anxiety, and Stress Disorders   150
Pain Disorders   151
Anxiety Disorders   166
Conclusions   187
BACB Task List (5th edition)   194

7. Neurological Disorders   197
Essential Tremor   197
Tourette's Syndrome   211
Huntington's Disease   213
Traumatic Brain Injury   214
Conclusions   220
BACB Task List (5th edition)   223

8. Where do we go from here?   226
Basic Research Questions   226

Questions of Clinical Significance   228
The Clinician as Researcher   231
Conclusions   232
BACB Task List (5th edition)   234

Appendices
A. Tension Self-Report Rating and Home Practice Record   237
B. States of Arousal and Relaxation Scale   238
C. Behavioral Relaxation Scale   241
D. Acquisition Training Protocol for Use with Trainers   242
E. Pre-post Relaxation Distress Rating Scale   245
F. Contract for Maintaining Behavior Change   246
G. Residential BRT Checklist   247
H. Caregiver Reclined Relaxed Behavior Rating Form   248
I. Reclined Relaxed BRT Acquisition Training Protocol   249
J. Written Criterion Tests for Behavioral Relaxation Scale Observers   250

Name Index   253
Subject Index   257

ABOUT THE AUTHORS

Duane A. Lundervold is a Professor and the Coordinator of the Master of Science in Behavior Analysis program at the University of Central Missouri (UCM). Duane is a graduate of Southern Illinois University-Carbondale and the Rehabilitation Institute. He is a Board Certified Behavior Analyst–Doctoral level (BCBA–D) and a Licensed Professional Counselor (Missouri, Wisconsin). He has served as editor of *Behavior Analysis: Research and Practice* published by the American Psychological Association. While at UCM, he and his students have conducted basic and applied research related to behavioral relaxation training (BRT), mindfulness, behavioral activation treatment for pain, essential tremor, and Parkinson's disease. Dr. Lundervold also has an appointment in the Department of Neuroscience at Saint Luke's Hospital-Kansas City and is a member of Plaza Primary Care and Geriatrics, a multi-specialty medical practice also located in Kansas City.

Duane received his early training in behavior analysis at the University of Wisconsin-Eau Claire, where Dr. Kenneth D. McIntire opened the door of his comparative experimental analysis of behavior laboratory and to a new world.

Roger Poppen is Professor Emeritus of the Behavior Analysis and Therapy Program at Southern Illinois University-Carbondale. He received his PhD in psychology from Stanford University. Roger is the author of the biography, *Joseph Wolpe, Key Figures in Psychotherapy* (1996), and the first and second editions of *Behavioral Relaxation Training and Assessment* (1988, 1996). While at SIU-C he served as coordinator of the Behavior Analysis program and on the editorial board of *Behavior Therapy and Experimental Psychiatry*. He and his students were responsible for the first-generation development and evaluation of behavioral relaxation training. He currently resides in Saint Louis, Missouri where he spends time with Bruno, terrier extraordinaire, traveling, enjoying his children and grandchildren, and writing.

John M. Guercio is Clinical Director of Behavior Analysis and Therapy services at Benchmark Human Services in Saint Louis, Missouri. Dr. Guercio is a Board Certified Behavior Analyst-Doctoral level, Missouri Licensed Behavior Analyst, and Certified Brain Injury Specialist Trainer. He has also served as past president of the Missouri Association for Behavior Analysis. John received his graduate training at Southern Illinois University-Carbondale, and has spent much of his career researching effective staff training protocols and behavioral intervention strategies for staff and participants in treatment settings with severe aggressive behavior. He has given more than 100 presentations at behavioral conferences, authored and/or co-authored over 50 articles in peer reviewed journals, and written several book chapters related to the treatment of intensive behavioral issues.

Foreword

Peter Sturmey, Ph.D
City University of New York

Let me begin with a confession of bias: I am a great fan of relaxation training. It was the only clinical skill that I was taught in a British clinical psychology program many years ago; everything else was left to chance. It was taught badly and incompletely, and no one observed me teaching patients to use it: They just believed me when I said I did it well.

Nevertheless, I use relaxation a lot in my life. As an over-enthusiastic graduate student, I used to get pain in my left shoulder and tension headaches when studying. After learning relaxation training, I became aware that I placed my left hand under the desk and, over the course of a couple of hours, would press harder and harder. Once I noticed this, I placed my hand on the desktop and relaxed with a few deep breaths. I have not had shoulder pain or tension headaches for nearly 40 years. In another personal application, I developed a version of relaxation for singing classical music by identifying all the muscles involved in singing and using a modified version of progressive relaxation training for those muscles. I often use relaxation when I stress out, when learning diving, or before giving a speech in front of a large unfamiliar audience. I try to use it when driving in New York City, but so far with limited success; perhaps I should not be relaxed in that situation.

Many forms of relaxation are cultural practices that we all are familiar with: "Take a deep breath," "Just calm down." And there are plenty of books and other media on meditation, yoga, prayer, and mindfulness, which are all practices that involve relaxation in some form. So why do we need another book on relaxation training?

The first and most important feature of this volume is that it takes a distinct conceptual approach to relaxation training, namely applied behavior analysis. This is both more conceptually consistent and technological than other methods. The authors define relaxed and non-relaxed behavior clearly and provide images of what relaxation looks like. They distinguish acquisition of relaxation skills from proficient performance, generalization, and maintenance. Methods to train observers to measure relaxation are spelled out, evaluated and shown to be reliable. And methods of training practitioners to correctly use relaxation training also are clearly presented, using behavioral skills training. In terms of conceptual consistency and empirical rigor, this volume offers a powerful alternative to approaches typical of clinical psychology and other mental health disciplines.

Second, these authors have worked in an unusually wide range of settings and with a wide range of populations, as evidenced in the Chapter headings, as well with as a wide range of ages, from children to seniors. This volume provides numerous and diverse practical examples of the application of standardized relaxation training, along with modifications for individuals with special needs, that readers will find very helpful in their research and applied work. In addition, practitioners will benefit from the numerous appendices of helpful forms. The authors are dedicated to helping people. They are empiricists, and their case studies are full of meaningful data. Moreover, their ethical and humane concern for their fellow humans is evident throughout the book.

Third, the authors' years of applied and research work shines through. This volume represents the accumulation of many years of work of three highly experienced researcher-practitioners. For example, when considering the question of evidence-based practice, the evidence is varied when considered disorder by disorder. These authors correctly acknowledge both the areas where positive evidence has accumulated and areas where much more needs to be done.

At the end, I was impressed with all that these authors, and other researchers in the field of relaxation training, have achieved. I wondered as to how does relaxation training fit into an overall self-managed life. Stress is something all of us deal with, and the place of relaxation training in a self-managed life will be different for each of us. A second thought was how future researchers can address large-scale dissemination of such a widely useful skill set. Can we make this material readily available on the Internet and digital platforms for everyone to use? If parents can teach their children to relax, can piano teachers, life coaches and work supervisors do the same on a large scale? How can this effective technology be made widely accessible to all that might need it?

We should all thank Duane A. Lundervold, Roger Poppen, and John M. Guercio for putting together this concise, wonderful and thoughtful volume that many clinicians will find to be a useful and practical guide to their applied work.

—Peter Sturmey, Ph.D.,
Professor, Department of Psychology,
The City University of New York

Chapter 1
Stress and Coping

TWO CASE STUDIES

Janice

Janice was devastated. At age sixty-nine, her "golden years" had turned to ashes. As a stay-at-home mom, she had cared for her children and managed the household. Financial matters were her husband's responsibility. Although she used the checkbook and credit cards, where the money came from and how much was in the bank was not her concern. Then her husband, a physician, had dropped the bomb; he told her the bank had called in the loan on his business and he didn't know how he was going to cover it. "Oh no," she thought, "we're going to lose everything: our house, our cars, our life savings, and, of course, his practice. What will our children think, our friends and neighbors? We are ruined."

The ensuing week was unbearable. During the day she felt exhausted and irritable, sometimes bursting into tears. At night, she would fall asleep for a short time, only to awaken and lie in bed plagued by thoughts of economic catastrophe, personal failure, and embarrassment. Mornings were awful, anxiety coming in waves. Tension built throughout the day as time for her husband's homecoming approached. But they couldn't talk, or else they lapsed into arguments and recriminations.

Janice* felt totally out of control of her life, and finally made an appointment with her primary care doctor, who was part of an integrated medical practice. She was prescribed anxiolytic and antidepressant medication and

---

*All of the individuals described in the clinical and research examples provided consent to take part in the research or allow use of their data. All projects were approved by the relevant institutional review board.

was referred to behavioral medicine services, carried out by the first author (DAL).

The initial interview established rapport, explored her "values for living," and revealed the context for her problematic behavior. The therapist explained that one's "values" serve as guides for action, and behavior that conflicts with these values causes distress. Janice's values included living a healthy life, which for her meant minimizing reliance on medications for panic relief, and having a good marital relationship.

DAL explained how the threat of bankruptcy was a powerful stressful event that negatively affected her coping abilities and her relationship with her husband. Stressors trigger dysfunctional thinking, unpleasant physiological reactions, and maladaptive avoidance responses. Janice wanted her suffering to go away without medication, but this would require her to discover stress triggers and to learn effective ways of coping with them. She agreed to an action plan with the ultimate goal of responding adaptively to the threats facing her.

Assessment via the Geriatric Depression Scale-15 (GDS-15)[1] and the Geriatric Anxiety Inventory (GAI)[2] indicated significant dysphoria. Worrisome covert self-talk (e.g., "We'll lose everything," "We're ruined") was identified as a key target behavior. Such thoughts were accompanied by severe distress. To measure the frequency and intensity of her stress responses and the events triggering them, Janice was instructed in the use of self-recording in her home environment. She noted the time and circumstances in which she engaged in negative self-talk, and rated the intensity of her negative feelings on a Subjective Units of Disturbance (SUD) Scale.[3] The following week, her self-recorded data revealed that worry behavior occurred with high frequency in the morning, as time for mail delivery approached, and in anticipation of her husband's arrival home after work.

To counteract aversive arousal, Janice was taught to relax using Behavioral Relaxation Training (BRT). She easily learned the relaxed postures in both reclined and upright sitting positions and reported feelings of calmness and that her "mind was not filled with worry" while relaxed. At home, Janice engaged in relaxation during those times and circumstances that previously had evoked worrisome self-talk and anxious arousal. She reported marked decreases in frequency of ruminative thinking and SUD ratings. Scores on the GDS-15 and GAI improved markedly. She found that the effect of relaxation was equal to the anxiolytic medication and ceased using it, meeting another of her treatment goals. Moreover, her sleep improved as did interactions with her husband. No change in the family's financial situation had occurred, so Janice needed to continue to use her relaxation skills to cope with this stressor. But she no longer magnified its effects by incessant worry.

Larry

Larry, a forty-two-year-old man diagnosed with autism spectrum disorder (ASD), was removed from his home at age twenty when his family could no longer tolerate his extreme agitation and physical aggression. He spent the next two decades in and out of various state institutions, culminating in placement in a forensic unit. His aggressive behavior there was described as unmanageable. Staff routinely wore kickboxing pads to deflect his blows. His records indicated that some staff had suffered broken noses. He had a history of property destruction during public outings, where, for example, he flipped over tables in restaurants and threw food containers on the floor. Police had to be called on several occasions. He also engaged in self-injurious behavior.

Shortly after his forty-first birthday, Larry was transferred to a community-based residential facility where JMG was a consultant. Several direct and indirect assessment procedures were employed to determine situations likely to trigger Larry's aggressive behavior as well as the consequences of his actions. These included the Functional Assessment Screening Tool (FAST), Questions About Behavioral Function (QABF), and the Functional Analysis Inventory (FAI).[4]

The goal of each of these indirect assessment instruments was to gather information on the functions of maladaptive behavior. Staff were trained in direct behavioral observation and event recording, as well as descriptive functional assessment procedures. Results indicated that the primary function of Larry's aggressive behavior was to gain staff attention. Outbursts were more likely when favorite staff members were not present or were leaving during change of shift. Larry reported that he missed his family and feeling lonely was upsetting to him. Conversely, feeling crowded by other residents was also stressful and could trigger aggressive behavior. Larry's limited verbal skills prevented him from communicating when he felt stressed, lonely, or upset.

To cope with provocative situations and upset feelings, Larry was taught relaxation using BRT. In particular, he was taught to recognize tense muscles and increased breathing rate in upsetting situations, such as shift changes, and to engage in relaxed behavior. In addition, staff was trained to prompt Larry to use his relaxation skills and to give him positive attention when he did so. Larry rapidly learned the relaxed postures and was able to implement them as needed during the day. The frequency of aggressive actions toward others, self-injurious behavior, and instances of property destruction decreased markedly during and after the two-year implementation of the relaxation program.

Summary

Janice and Larry are two markedly different people and appear to have very different problems. Janice, threatened by financial ruin, reacts with crippling anxiety. Larry, burdened by ASD, faces both social isolation and crowding in an institutional setting and responds with aggressive outbursts. Yet, there is a common element. Both find themselves in an ongoing, demanding situation for which they have no adequate coping skills. This state of affairs arouses anxiety in Janice and anger in Larry. Janice deals with anxiety by ruminative worry, which solves nothing and only makes matters worse. Larry lashes out at others in his environment, which serves to maintain his institutional confinement. They are trapped.

STRESS

Fight-or-flight is a concept introduced by Walter B. Cannon early in the twentieth century.[5] He discovered the biological changes occurring within an animal that enhance its chances of survival when confronted with threatening circumstances. For example, a cat confronted with a barking dog undergoes increased secretion of adrenaline, increased heart and respiration rate, increased blood flow to skeletal muscles, decreased blood flow to skin and digestive organs, pupillary dilation, and piloerection. These changes are mediated by arousal of the sympathetic branch of the autonomic nervous system. Cannon also developed the concept of *homeostasis*.[6] When the threat passes, the parasympathetic branch aids in reversing arousal; the animal calms down and is able to engage in restorative behavior, such as eating, digestion, or sexual activity, depending on circumstances. Thus, the two branches of the autonomic nervous system engage in a process of dynamic regulation, preparing the animal to deal with the exigencies of daily life.

Cannon extrapolated these concepts to human emotions and illness. In an address to medical colleagues in 1936, he noted how modern life had become so fast-paced and uncertain that people often were in a perpetual state of arousal, with little opportunity for homeostatic return to resting levels. He observed that participants no longer suffered from old-style "plagues and pestilences," but from "strains and stresses" of daily life. "It is not surprising, therefore, that fear and worry and hate can lead to harmful and profoundly disturbing consequences."[7] As prescient as his message was, several more decades and much more research were necessary before the idea gained wide currency.

Hans Selye is credited with developing the concept of *stress* as it is currently viewed in relation to human health problems.[8] Beginning in the 1930's, Selye conducted a series of studies on laboratory rodents in which he subjected them to biochemical agents that made them ill, or environmental demands that taxed their limits of endurance. Despite the variety of circumstances, he discovered a common biological response which he first termed the *General Adaptation Syndrome* and later the *stress response*.[9] He differentiated *acute stress*, in which the demanding situation is time-limited or amenable to a solution (corresponding to Cannon's fight-or-flight response), from *chronic stress*, which ensued when there is no escape. In the former circumstances, biological arousal is beneficial, in that it equips the organism to deal with the situation, whereas the latter results in illness or death. Like Cannon, Selye remained an animal researcher, but late in his career, he reviewed the work of others that demonstrated the effects of stress on human health.[10]

Despite the admonitions of Cannon and Selye to their medical colleagues concerning the importance of disorders due to chronic stress, as compared to acute disorders that arise from injury or infection, traditional medicine could only provide the usual interventions—surgery, medication, and perhaps advice on lifestyle change. This began to change in the 1970s with the emergence of the interdisciplinary field of *behavioral medicine*. In 1977, the Yale Conference on Behavioral Medicine brought together an eminent group of behavioral and biomedical scientists to develop a definition of the scope and boundaries of this burgeoning interdisciplinary field.[11] They recognized that behavioral concepts and techniques were applicable to a wide range of medical problems, including what have come to be called stress-related disorders, such as headache (tension and migraine), hypertension and other cardiovascular diseases, and various gastrointestinal disorders such as irritable bowel syndrome. In addition, chronic biomedical conditions, such as Crohn's disease, Parkinson's disease, chronic back pain, ASD, intellectual disability, and chemotherapy regimens for cancer, can cause stress that serves to exacerbate the participant's suffering.

ANXIETY

Anxiety can be defined as a particular class of stress response that is characterized by negative affect, increased arousal, and attempts to escape or avoid upsetting situations. Sufferers describe feelings of fear and apprehension that some overwhelming circumstance may befall them. To the extent they are able to identify those circumstances, anxiety sufferers avoid them. Often it is the anxious feelings themselves that people seek to escape or avoid by means of mood-altering drugs such as nicotine, alcohol, or anxiolytic medication. This, in turn, can lead to even more problems with which the individual must cope.

Basic Research on Anxiety

The psychological concept of anxiety became popular early in the twentieth century from the psychoanalytic theory of Sigmund Freud.[12] In this theory, neurotic anxiety arises from conflict between the libidinous urges of the id and repression by the superego. Psychoanalytic therapy aimed at relieving conflict by uncovering these hidden urges through indirect methods such as free-association and dream interpretation.

The idea of conflict between excitatory and inhibitory unconscious mental forces influenced early laboratory research. Ivan Pavlov,[13] in the course of his pioneering studies of conditioned reflexes, found that certain procedures resulted in what he termed "experimental neurosis," characterized by agitated behavior and loss of previously learned responses. In his well-known respondent conditioning paradigm with dogs, a meat pellet, employed as the unconditioned stimulus (US), elicits salivation (unconditioned response, or UR). An auditory signal (conditioned stimulus, or CS) that routinely precedes the US eventually comes to elicit salivation (conditioned response, or CR) on trials when the US is omitted. But if a mild aversive stimulus, such as a low amperage electric shock is used as the CS, with food as the US, a salivation CR may be learned, but soon disappears, accompanied by the dog resisting being put in the experimental apparatus and other "neurotic" behavior. Pavlov attributed this to a "clash" between excitatory and inhibitory cortical states induced by the positive (food) and negative (shock) stimuli.

Jules Masserman[14] followed up this idea in experiments with cats trained to lift the lid of a food box with their paws when an auditory or visual stimulus was presented. This differs from the Pavlovian respondent conditioning paradigm in that a motor response is required to obtain the food. In this case, the auditory stimulus serves a discriminative function (discriminative stimulus or S^D) that signals when the food (reinforcing stimulus or S^{R+}) is available. The animal then manipulates its environment to obtain the food. This is termed *instrumental* or *operant conditioning*. Respondent conditioning occurs concurrently with the auditory signal becoming a CS for salivation (CR, not measured) elicited by the food (US). Masserman then introduced conflict by shocking the animal as it lifted the lid of the food box. He attributed the resulting upset to conflict between approach and avoidance drive states.

Joseph Wolpe[15] tested the necessity of the conflict hypothesis by repeating the Masserman procedure with two groups of cats. One group received the auditory signal and was trained to engage in eating, and then was shocked while eating; another group simply received the signal, followed by shock. Both groups of cats became equally agitated and refused food in the experimental chamber. Wolpe concluded that anxiety had been acquired according to Pavlovian conditioning principles. The auditory signal (and cage) functioned as a CS, the shock was the US, fear arousal to the shock was the UR, and anxiety—anticipatory arousal—was the CR. Conflict was irrelevant.

As Pavlov, Masserman, and other researchers noted, conditioned anxiety is markedly resistant to standard respondent extinction procedures, in which the CS is presented without the US. Wolpe's major contribution was to develop a method to overcome anxiety in his experimental subjects, which he then extrapolated to treat human anxiety disorders.[16] Wolpe's pioneering efforts provide the foundation for current evidence-based cognitive-behavioral treatment programs for anxiety disorders.

Clinical Diagnosis of Anxiety

While most people experience anxiety in one form or another, to be classified as a disorder the condition must cause significant distress and impair the person's functioning in daily life.[17] It has been estimated that around thirty percent of adults living in the United States have suffered from an anxiety disorder at some point in their lives that meets clinical criteria.[18] Some of these disorders, categorized in terms of their eliciting events, are listed below.

POST-TRAUMATIC-STRESS-DISORDER (PTSD). PTSD bears the closest resemblance to the conditioned anxiety studied by animal researchers. An individual experiences extreme fear in a life-threatening circumstance; for example, a soldier in a combat setting. Later, some stimulus related to that experience, such as the sound of glass breaking or a car backfiring, can trigger a full-blown panic response. (It was his study and treatment of "shell shocked" soldiers in the First World War that led to Joseph Wolpe's interest in the role of Pavlovian conditioning in anxiety acquisition.)[19] A person with PTSD tends to avoid novel or unfamiliar settings where an unexpected stimulus may set off an anxiety attack.

Specific Phobias

For specific phobias, such as fear of heights, snakes, or spiders, the connection to the CS is obvious. In some cases, the person may have suffered a traumatic respondent conditioning episode, such as being bitten by a dog. But in many other instances, the phobic person has never had direct aversive contact with the dreaded stimulus; the US may be purely imaginal, as when the person visualizes falling or being bitten. In other cases, the person can acquire the fear through observation as part of the respondent conditioning process; for example, a child observes a parent exhibiting fear (US) of a mouse (CS). People with phobias avoid contact with the CS; for example, an arachnophobe (fearful of spiders) is unlikely to take a walk in the woods and a claustrophobe (fearful of closed spaces) may take the stairs rather than an elevator.

SOCIAL PHOBIA. People with social phobia fear that others will negatively evaluate or ridicule their appearance or performance. This may arise from an actual humiliating experience or, as with specific phobias, the person may imagine such a horrifying event. People with social fears typically avoid participation in classroom or workplace discussions and are hesitant about meeting new people.

PANIC DISORDER. In panic disorder, a triggering stimulus is not obvious. A panic attack is characterized by racing heart, difficulty breathing, dizziness or faintness, feeling hot flashes or chills—in other words, a full-blown fight-or-flight response. This is highly aversive and the person experiences it as a complete loss of control, going crazy or impending death. Panic sufferers tend to have a heightened awareness of bodily sensations, such as heart rate, which can then serve as a CS for a full-blown attack. They develop a "fear of fear." Since there is no identifiable external environmental CS, many people with this disorder avoid situations where there is no easy escape or no trusted person who could provide care should an attack occur, thus limiting their mobility and independence. This condition is known as *agoraphobia*.

GENERALIZED ANXIETY DISORDER. This condition is characterized by a plethora of daily life events that evoke anxious arousal and worry. Rather than an overwhelming episode, as in panic disorder, the person suffers continual low-level arousal. And since the upsetting cues are present throughout the day, there is little chance of escape or avoidance. Janice, whom we met at the beginning of this chapter, is a good example.

ANGER

If anxiety is the emotional accompaniment to the *flight* portion of the stress response, anger is the emotional component of the *fight* reaction. Anger can be regarded as an emotional reaction to environmental events that impose or threaten injury or loss, a reaction which mediates aggressive behavior. Cannon focused on the pattern of physiologic arousal that facilitates the animal's survival rather than its subjective feelings. Recall the hissing, claws-baring cat facing a barking dog, prepared to attack if the dog ventures too close. Aggressive behavior has the evolutionary function of damaging the opponent or driving it away, thus increasing chances of prevailing in combat.

In human social situations, where direct physical altercations are usually prohibited, aggression may be expressed verbally, through threats and curses, or by assaulting the environment, such as slamming a door, or taken out on an innocent bystander, such as yelling at one's spouse. In addition, there are circumstances where aggressive behavior may be prized without regard to its precursor emotions. For example, boxing, wrestling, and other martial arts are regulated forms of aggression in which the combatants may or may not be angry with each other, but it is easy to see how such feelings could arise. Boxers at weigh-in, before a match, often adopt an angry mien and confront each other as much as possible without actually coming to blows.

Basic Research on Anger

Perhaps the earliest and most influential analyses of aggression was presented by a group of researchers at Yale University in 1939.[20,21] They focused on *frustration*, which refers to the procedure of blocking or thwarting goal-directed behavior. To be frustrated is to be engaged in a task that routinely pays off (is reinforced), but then the expected outcome does not occur. Think of the vending machine that regularly dispenses candy, but one time when you put your money in and pull the handle, nothing happens. An aggressive response, such as pounding on the front of the machine or kicking it, is quite common. Frustration refers to the feeling one has in such a circumstance. The aggressive response may be effective in freeing up a jammed candy bar, but in most instances, it has no obvious beneficial consequences.

Berkowitz[21,22] provides a comprehensive review of research and theory on the relationship between frustration, aggression, and anger in humans. Research took the form of surveys, in which people reported occasions on which they became angry or aggressive, and laboratory experiments, where subjects (usually college students) working on a task were prevented from completing it and attaining a reward. Anger was measured by self-report, penalties which the subjects exacted on the perceived agent of frustration or innocent bystanders, and by changes in relevant physiological systems. Factors such as perceived fairness/unfairness of the interruption and the personal significance of the goal can influence the probability or magnitude of the anger response. But, Berkowitz concluded, there is one basic feature of all anger-evoking situations, and that is aversiveness. Generally speaking, the more aversive the circumstances, the stronger or more likely the anger response. Perceived arbitrariness, or malice of the thwarting agent, or importance of the blocked reward, serve to make the frustrating situation more aversive.

Considering frustration to be aversive connects it to the large amount of research on *pain-elicited* aggression (reviewed by Ulrich[23]). Laboratory experimentation has shown that periodic, unavoidable electric shock elicits fighting behavior in pairs of rats or pigeons, and biting responses in monkeys. Systematic relationships are found between latency or probability of fighting and the intensity, frequency, and duration of shock. Aggressive behavior can be conditioned to stimuli paired with shock in a respondent conditioning paradigm. Also, animals can learn an operant response that provides them with a target for aggression during periods of electric shock. Animals will also attack a target, or learn a response that provides a target to attack, during periods of extinction of positively reinforced behavior. Extinction consists of withholding regularly scheduled reinforcers, and thus can be considered to be a frustration procedure, further demonstrating the aversive nature of frustration.

It is not difficult to think of everyday experiences in which a painful stimulus, such as hitting one's thumb with a hammer, will elicit angry verbal aggression (cursing) or physical lashing out. In research with human subjects, aversive environments, while not as explicitly intense as electric shock or a hammer blow, have been shown to produce or heighten anger. Persons exposed to either uncomfortably warm or cold environments expressed anger and hostility toward a peer, even though that person had nothing to do with their discomfort.[24] Other research has shown that cigarette smoke and foul odors heighten expressions of hostility or punishments delivered to another person.[25]

At its core, anger is an automatic response to an aversive situation, with characteristic autonomic and overt behavioral components geared toward attack on the aversive agent or a convenient bystander.[26] Humans, as a result of social learning, may also engage in cognitive appraisal of the justification or motivation of the aversive agent, as well as the consequences of aggression. Self-talk (verbal behavior) can affect the likelihood or magnitude of the aggressive response, but is not an essential component. Indeed, it is the reflexive lashing out, without consideration of situation or consequences, that gets people in trouble and is the target for intervention.

Clinical Diagnosis of Anger

In contrast to the many guises of anxiety disorder, only one type of anger disorder is recognized by the *Diagnostic and Statistical Manual of Mental Dis-*

orders-5, namely intermittent explosive disorder (IED).[27] This is a sudden aggressive outburst, verbal and/or physical, entirely disproportionate to the circumstances in which it occurs. Lifetime adult prevalence estimates are about seven percent, although some researchers contend it is understudied and under-diagnosed.[28,29]

IED has been shown to be related to various markers of severe criminal behavior among federal prisoners.[30] Even at subclinical levels, it is obvious how angry outbursts impair functioning in home, school, and work settings. In addition, anger has been shown to increase risk of coronary heart disease.[31,32]

Novaco[33] pioneered the development of evidence-based procedures, including relaxation training, used in the treatment of anger. Numerous studies have been conducted demonstrating the utility of relaxation as part of a treatment package or as a stand-alone treatment[34-37] for individuals with problems with anger and aggression, or with anger-related health problems.[38,39] Lindsay and colleagues[40] demonstrated that with appropriate instruction, individuals with intellectual disabilities could learn to reliably describe the occurrence of anger. They have also shown that relaxation is a functional replacement behavior. Skills in relaxation provide an individual with a developmental disability greater autonomy, independence, self-determination and self-control. The case of Larry is an excellent example.

CONCLUSIONS

Stress places demands upon individuals that severely test their coping abilities. If not dealt with effectively, stress can exacerbate medical illnesses such as cardiovascular disorders, gastrointestinal disorders, headache and other types of pain, and lowered immune system functioning. Stress exacts an emotional toll in terms of anxiety, anger, and depression. People often deal with stress by using psychoactive substances such as alcohol, nicotine, or cannabis, as well as a host of prescription and over-the-counter medications. These may produce short-term benefits, but long-term use can result in decreased effectiveness as well as additional problems such as drug-dependency or adverse side-effects.

Relaxation is an essentially benign state that reduces or rebalances the physiological and psychological arousal that characterizes stress. It provides a means of coping, and facilitates learning additional coping skills, to deal with upsetting situations. The following chapter discusses relaxation in general and provides a behavioral framework to show its mechanism of action for overcoming stress and its unfortunate consequences.

REFERENCES

[1]Sheikh, J. I. & Yesavage, J. A. (1986). Geriatric Depression Scale (GDS). Recent evidence and development of a shorter version. In T. L. Brink (Ed.), *Clinical Gerontology: A Guide to Assessment and Intervention* (pp. 165–173). NY: The HaworthPress, Inc.

[2]Pachana, N. A., Byrne, G. J., Siddle, H., Koloski, N., Harley, E., & Arnold, E. (2007). Development and validation of the Geriatric Anxiety Inventory. *International Psychogeriatrics, 19,* 103–14.

[3]Wolpe, J. & Lazarus, A. A. (1966). *Behavior therapy techniques: A guide to the treatment of neurosis.* NY: Pergamon.

[4]Zaja, R. H., Moore, L., Van Ingen, D. J., & Rojahn, J. (2011). Psychometric comparison of the functional assessment instruments QABF, FAI and FAST for self-injurious, stereotypic and aggressive/destructive behavior. *Journal of Applied Research in Intellectual Disabilities, 24,* 18–28.

[5]Cannon, W. B. (1915). *Bodily changes in pain, hunger, fear and rage: An account of recent researches into the function of emotional excitement.* NY: Appleton-Century-Crofts.

[6]Goldstein, D. (May 16, 2009). *Walter Cannon: Homeostasis, the Fight-or-Flight Response, the sympathoadrenal system, and the wisdom of the body.* Retrieved January 8, 2016 from http://www.brainimmune.com/walter-cannon-homeostasis-the-fight-or-flight-response-the-sympathoadrenal-system-and-the-wisdom-of-the-body/

[7]Cannon, W. B. (1936). *The Role of Emotion in Disease.* Convocation Oration delivered to the Twentieth Annual Session of the American College of Physicians.

[8]Szabo, S., Tache, Y., & Somogyi, A. (2012). The legacy of Hans Selye and the origins of stress research: A retrospective 75 years after his landmark brief "Letter to the Editor" of Nature. *Stress, 15*(5), 472–478.

[9]Selye, H. (1956). *The stress of life.* McGraw Hill. New York: New York.

[10]Selye, H. (1976). *Stress in health and disease.* Boston: Butterworth.

[11]Schwarz, G. E. & Weiss, S. M. (1977). *Proceedings of the Yale Conference of Behavioral Medicine.* U.S. Department of Health, Education, and Welfare, DHEW Publication No. (NIH) 78–1424.

[12]Freud, S. (1923). *The Ego and the Id.* NY: W.W. Norton & Co.

[13]Pavlov, I. (1927). *Conditioned reflexes: An investigation of the physiological activity of the cerebral cortex.* London: Oxford University Press.

[14]Masserman, J. (1943). *Behavior and neurosis.* Chicago: University of Chicago Press.

[15]Wolpe, J. (1952). Objective psychotherapy for neuroses. *South African Medical Journal, 26,* 825–829.

[16]Wolpe, J. (1958). *Psychotherapy by reciprocal inhibition.* Stanford, CA: Stanford University Press.

[17]*Diagnostic and Statistical Manual of Mental Disorders, 5th ed.* (2013). Arlington, VA: American Psychiatric Publishing.

[18]*Any anxiety disorder.* Retrieved February 14, 2019 from https://www.nimh.nih.gov/health/statistics/any-anxiety-disorder.shtml#part_155094

[19]Poppen, R. (2001). Joseph Wolpe: Challenger and champion for Behavior Therapy. In W.T. O'Donohue, D. A. Henderson, S.C. Hayes, J.E. Fisher, & L.J. Hayes (Eds.), *A history of the behavioral therapies: Founders personal stories* (pp. 39–58).

[20]Dollard, J., Doob, L., Miller, N., Mowrer, O., & Sears, R. (1939). *Frustration and aggression*. New Haven, CT: Yale University Press.

[21]Berkowitz, L. (1989). Frustration-aggression hypothesis: Examination and reformulation. *Psychological Bulletin, 106*, 59–73.

[22]Berkowitz, L. & Harmon-Jones, E. (2004). Toward and understanding of the determinants of anger. *Emotion, 4*, 107–130. doi: 10.1037/1528-3542.4.2.107

[23]Ulrich, R. (1966). Pain as a cause of aggression. *American Zoologist, 6*, 643–662.

[24]Anderson, C. A. & Anderson, K. B. (1998). Temperature and aggression: Paradox, controversy, and a (fairly) clear picture. In R. G. Geen & E. Donnerstein (Eds.), *Human aggression: Theories, research, and implications for social policy* (pp. 247–298). San Diego, CA: Academic Press.

[25]Berkowitz, L. (1983). Aversively stimulated aggression: Some parallels and differences in research with animals and humans. *American Psychologist, 38*, 1135–1144.

[26]Berkowitz, L. (2012). A different view of anger: The cognitive-neoassociation conception of the relation of anger to aggression. *Aggressive Behavior, 38*, 322–333. https://doi.org/10.1002/ab.21432

[27]*Intermittent Explosive Disorder DSM–5 312.34*. Retrieved on February 14, 2019 from (F63.81)https://www.theravive.com/therapedia/intermittent-explosive-disorder-dsm--5-312.34-(f63.81)

[28]*Intermittent Explosive Disorder Affects Up To 16 Million Americans*. Retrieved on February 14, 2019 from https://www.sciencedaily.com/releases/2006/06/060606092346.htm

[29]McLaughlin, K. A., Green, J., Hwang, I., Sampson, N. A., Zaslavsky, A. M., & Kessler, R. C. (2012) Intermittent explosive disorder in the National Comorbidity Survey Replication Adolescent Supplement. *Archives of General Psychiatry, 69*(11), 1131–1139

[30]DeLisi, M., Elbert, M., Caropreso, D., Tahja, K., Heinrichs, T., & Drury, A. (2017). Criminally explosive: Intermittent explosive disorder, Criminal careers, and psychopathology among federal correctional participants. *International Journal of Forensic Mental Health, 16*(4), 293–303. doi: 10.1080/14999013.2017.1365782

[31]Chida, Y. & Steptoe, A. (2009). The association of anger and hostility with future coronary heart disease. A meta-analytic review of prospective evidence. *Journal of the American College of Cardiology, 53*(11), 936–46. doi: 10.1016/j.jacc.2008.11.044.

[32]Mostofsky, E., Penner, E. A., & Mittleman, M. A. (2014). Outbursts of anger as a trigger of acute cardiovascular events: a systematic review and meta-analysis. *European Heart Journal, 35*(21), 1404–10. doi: 10.1093/eurheartj/ehu033.

[33]Novaco, R. W. (1976). Treatment of chronic anger through cognitive and relaxation controls. *Journal of Consulting and Clinical Psychology, 44*(4), 681. http://dx.doi.org/10.1037/0022-006X.44.4.681

[34]Glancy, G., & Saini, M. (2005). An evidenced-based review of psychological treatments for anger and aggression. *Brief Treatment and Crisis Intervention, 5*, 229–248.

[35]Taylor, J. L., Novaco, R. W., Gillmer, B. T., Robertson, A., & Thorne, I. (2005). Individual cognitive-behavioral anger treatment for people with mild-borderline intellectual disabilities and histories of aggression: A controlled trial. *British Journal of Clinical Psychology, 44*, 367–382. doi:10.1348/014466505X29990

[36]Tafrate, R.C. (1995). Evaluation of treatment strategies for adult anger. In H. Kassinove (Ed.), *Anger disorders* (pp. 109–129). Washington, DC: Taylor & Francis.

[37]Beck, R., & Fernandez, E. (1998). Cognitive-behavioral therapy in the treatment of anger: A meta-analysis. *Cognitive Therapy and Research, 22,* 63–74.

[38]Stahl, J. E., Dossett, M. L., LaJoie, A. S., Denninger, J. W., Mehta, D. H., Goldman, R., et al. (2015). Relaxation response and resiliency training and its effect on healthcare resource utilization. *PLoS ONE 10(10): e0140212.* doi:10.1371/journal.pone.0140212.

[39]Blumenthal, J. A., Jiang, W., Babyak, M. A., et al., (1997). Stress management and exercise training in cardiac participants with myocardial ischemia. Effects on prognosis and evaluation of mechanisms. *Archives of Internal Medicine, 157(19),* 2213–2223. doi:10.1001/archinte.1997.00440400063008

[40]Lindsay, W. R., Fee., M., Michie, A. M., & Heap. I. (1994). The effects of cue control relaxation on adults with severe mental retardation. *Research in Developmental Disabilities, 15,* 425–37.

[41]Williams, J. (1990) Helping people to relax in over stimulating environments. *Mental Handicap, 18,* 160–162.

Supplement
Behavior Analyst Certification Board 5th Edition Task List

Philosophical Underpinnings
A-2   Explain the philosophical assumptions underlying the science of behavior analysis (e.g., selectionism, determinism, empiricism, parsimony, pragmatism).
A-2   Explain the philosophical assumptions underlying the science of behavior analysis (e.g., selectionism, determinism, empiricism, parsimony, pragmatism).
A-3   Describe and explain behavior from the perspective of radical behaviorism.
A-4   Distinguish among behaviorism, the experimental analysis of behavior, applied behavior analysis, and professional practice guided by the science of behavior analysis.
A-3   Describe and explain behavior from the perspective of radical behaviorism.
A-5   Describe and define the dimensions of applied behavior analysis (Baer, Wolf, & Risley, 1968).

B. Concepts and Principles
B-1   Define and provide examples of behavior, response, and response class.
B-2   Define and provide examples of stimulus and stimulus class.
B-3   Define and provide examples of respondent and operant conditioning.
B-4   Define and provide examples of positive and negative reinforcement contingencies.
B-7   Define and provide examples of automatic and socially mediated contingencies.
B-13 Define and provide examples of rule-governed and contingency-shaped behavior.

C. Measurement, Data Display, and Interpretation
C-1   Establish operational definitions of behavior.
C-2   Distinguish among direct, indirect, and product measures of behavior.
C-3   Measure occurrence (e.g., frequency, rate, percentage).
C-4   Measure temporal dimensions of behavior (e.g., duration, latency, interresponse time).

C-5 Measure form and strength of behavior (e.g., topography, magnitude).
C-9 Select a measurement system to obtain representative data given the dimensions of behavior and the logistics of observing and recording.

D. Experimental Design
D-1 Distinguish between dependent and independent variables.

E. Ethics Behave in accordance with the Professional and Ethical Compliance Code for Behavior Analysts.
E-1 Responsible conduct of behavior analysts
E-2 Behavior analysts' responsibility to clients
E-3 Assessing behavior
E-4 Behavior analysts and the behavior-change program

F. Behavior Assessment
F-1 Review records and available data (e.g., educational, medical, historical) at the outset of the case.
F-2 Determine the need for behavior-analytic services.
F-3 Identify and prioritize socially significant behavior-change goals.
F-4 Conduct assessments of relevant skill strengths and deficits.
F-7 Conduct a descriptive assessment of problem behavior.
F-9 Interpret functional assessment data.

G. Behavior Change Procedures
G-1 Use positive and negative reinforcement procedures to strengthen behavior.
G-2 Use interventions based on motivating operations and discriminative stimuli.
G-3 Establish and use conditioned reinforcers.
G-4 Use stimulus and response prompts and fading (e.g., errorless, most-to-least, least-to-most, prompt delay, stimulus fading).
G-5 Use modeling and imitation training.
G-6 Use instructions and rules.
G-9 Use discrete-trial, free-operant, and naturalistic teaching arrangements.
G-14 Use reinforcement procedures to weaken behavior (e.g., DRA, FCT, DRO, DRL, NCR).
G-20 Use self-management strategies.

H. Selecting and Implementing Interventions

H-1 State intervention goals in observable and measurable terms.
H-2 Identify potential interventions based on assessment results and the best available scientific evidence.
H-3 Recommend intervention goals and strategies based on such factors as client preferences, supporting environments, risks, constraints, and social validity.
H-4 When a target behavior is to be decreased, select an acceptable alternative behavior to be established or increased.
H-5 Plan for possible unwanted effects when using reinforcement, extinction, and punishment procedures.
H-6 Monitor client progress and treatment integrity.
H-7 Make data-based decisions about the effectiveness of the intervention and the need for treatment revision.
H-8 Make data-based decisions about the need for ongoing services.
H-9 Collaborate with others who support and/or provide services to clients.

Chapter 2
Relaxation Training
An Overview

Relaxation training has been employed in treatments of stress and anxiety disorders for nearly a century. In that time, numerous training methods have emerged. At first glance, they appear to be grouped into two general categories based on the methods and targets of training, comprising an approximate mind/body dualism. Some procedures focus on physical training, which in turn produces mental effects. Others emphasize cognitive training, which are presumed to have effects on the body. The first section of this chapter describes various relaxation methods in terms of this mind/body heuristic.

The second section of this chapter considers theories of relaxation. Some emphasize its physiological aspects, others its mental nature. We propose a behavioral framework that subsumes these approaches, providing a common vocabulary for describing similarities and differences among methods.

Describing effects of relaxation training is matter of measurement. What happens as a result of training? The behavior analytic framework developed in this chapter provides the basis for measurement systems that are detailed in Chapter Three.

A BRIEF HISTORY AND DESCRIPTION OF RELAXATION TRAINING PROCEDURES

Physical Methods

PROGRESSIVE MUSCLE RELAXATION (PMR). In the 1920s, Edmund Jacobson, a Chicago physician and researcher, developed *progressive relaxation* as a method of treating participants suffering from "nervous tension." Symptoms as varied as fatigue, insomnia, headache, hypertension, ulcer, colitis, general anxiety, and specific phobias, were overcome by progressive relaxation.[1,2] Because of its focus on the skeletal musculature, this procedure has come to be called *Progressive Muscle Relaxation* (PMR), and this terminology will be employed in the rest of this book.

Jacobson taught participants to discriminate the sensations of tension and relaxation by instructing them to perform an action, such as making a fist, and to observe the tension in forearm and fingers; then to open the hand and note the change in feeling. Finer and finer discriminations were taught, so that the participant could detect the tension from the slight movement of a finger, say, and then any residual tension from no movement at all. This was repeated in a sequential, cumulative fashion for the various muscles throughout the body: face, neck, shoulders, chest, abdomen, back, legs, and feet. The participant reclined on a bed or chair that provided support while they relaxed their entire body. Training involved dozens of exercises carried out over many months. Between sessions, participants were instructed to practice an hour every day. Participants also were taught "differential relaxation," in which they learned to relax muscles that were not necessary in carrying out everyday tasks.

The goal of training was to attain as complete cessation of skeletal muscle activity as possible. To that end, Jacobson invented an "integrating neurovoltmeter," now called the electromyograph, allowing him to measure muscle action potentials down to the microvolt level.

Jacobson's career spanned four decades, during which he published descriptions of PMR applications for expectant mothers, businessmen, and psychiatric participants (*How to Relax and Have Your Baby*, 1959; *Tension Control for Businessmen*, 1963; *Modern Treatment of Tense Participants*, 1970).[3,4,5] But PMR got its biggest boost when Joseph Wolpe adapted it for use in a procedure specifically directed at phobic anxiety, a technique he termed *systematic desensitization*.[6] Wolpe drastically shortened the training time, finding that seven or eight sessions were sufficient to produce a state of relaxation that allowed the participant to remain calm when presented with attenuated forms of phobic stimuli. During desensitization training, aversive stimuli were presented in a hierarchy from low to high, over successive sessions, until the participant reported no anxiety to the top items. Differential relaxation also was encouraged, in which participants relaxed in their home or work environments, especially if phobic stimuli were encountered.

Systematic desensitization provided a bonanza for clinical researchers to investigate the parameters of the technique itself and to compare it with other procedures. Over the next three decades, thousands of studies were published. In this environment, PMR was standardized into a set number and sequence of exercises so that a specified "dose" could be administered to research subjects.[7] Beginning with individual muscles, later sessions collected them into muscle groups, like those of the legs or face. Instructions were delivered via audio recordings to further ensure equivalence across subjects, and participants could use the recordings for home practice. Other research employing PMR, for example, the biobehavioral treatment of headache, also uses recorded instructions.[8] While it is likely such attenuated procedures do not produce the profound relaxed state obtained by Jacobson, nonetheless, meaningful clinical improvements are widely found.

BEHAVIORAL RELAXATION TRAINING (BRT). Behavioral Relaxation Training has its roots in PMR. In the early 1980s, Don Schilling, a graduate student of author Roger Poppen, had difficulty teaching relaxation to a group of young adolescent boys with behavior disorders. He found that they were very good at tensing muscles but not so good at releasing the tension or noticing the differences between these two covert stimulus conditions. He wondered if there were ways to teach relaxation more directly. Accordingly, we set about to determine the target behaviors that characterize relaxation. That is, what does a completely relaxed person look like? And if we teach someone to look like that, are they relaxed according to other criteria?

Based on clinical experience, photographs provided in Jacobson's books, discussions with other professionals, and trial-and-error, we came up with a set of ten "relaxed behaviors" that could be taught by verbal description, modeling, and physical prompting.[9] Briefly, these are:

1. Head—supported by the chair cushion and straight with respect to body midline;
2. Eyes—lids closed smoothly and no motion of eyes beneath them;
3. Mouth—lips and teeth slightly parted;
4. Throat—motionless (e.g., no swallowing);
5. Shoulders—rounded, transect same horizontal plane, motionless;
6. Body—torso, hips, and legs symmetrical around midline, motionless;
7. Hands—resting on chair armrest or on thighs, palms down with fingers slightly curled;
8. Feet—heels on chair footrest with toes pointing in a V;
9. Quiet—no vocalizations or loud respiratory sounds;
10. Breathing—slow and regular. Training is typically carried out with the participant in a reclined position in a supportive chair (Reclined BRT), but modifications for an upright posture have been developed (Up-

right BRT, or UBRT). "Differential relaxation," based on the postures trained, as described by Jacobson, is also employed.

As with PMR, training proceeds in a sequential, cumulative manner, continuing until the participant reaches criterion—typically ninety percent or better of the relaxed behaviors during an observation period. Acquisition can be as short as a single session of less than an hour, or take several sessions for persons with special needs. Daily home practice is encouraged and additional training sessions may be necessary to insure mastery.

BRT contains a built-in assessment tool, the Behavioral Relaxation Scale (BRS), which is also useful for measuring outcomes with other training methods. The BRS is described more fully in Chapter Three. A full description of BRT—with details on training procedures and modifications—is provided in Chapter 4. Research on applications of BRT and comparisons with other methods are presented in subsequent chapters.

ELECTROMYOGRAPHIC BIOFEEDBACK (EMG-BF). As noted above, Jacobson invented an electronic device for measuring muscle activity in a circumscribed area. It can be said that if he had turned the instrument around so the participant could see the output of the device, he would have invented EMG biofeedback as well. Instead, it remained for Tom Budzynski to open the door for this line of inquiry and application.[10,11]

In this procedure, electrodes are placed on the skin surface above the muscles of interest and an auditory or visual signal that varies in proportion to muscle activity is provided. For example, in cases of tension headache, the frontalis muscles of the forehead are monitored and an auditory signal provided so that the participant can close their eyes and focus on the tone. Initially, the participant does not attend to muscle tension per se, but on the exteroceptive signal. By decreasing the pitch of the tone, the participant decreases muscle tension. Generalized relaxation may occur as well, due to the calming features of the training environment. In some training settings, EMG biofeedback is combined with additional relaxation methods to maximize clinical effectiveness.[8]

Individual training session duration is typically around a half-hour or less, because longer periods of focus on the signal can become tedious. Additional time may be spent discussing the participant's observations. Daily home practice is encouraged, with instructions to "do whatever you were doing to lower the tone in the office." A home-training device may be provided, but the ultimate goal of biofeedback is to teach participants to relax in the absence of the machine. To that end, as training progresses, the participant is instructed to attend to the muscle sensations related to the tone, and a threshold procedure may be employed, such that the signal turns off when tension is lowered below a certain value. Thus, the participant learns to relax in the absence of the signal. The number of sessions required to reach a desired level of relaxation varies among participants, but generally falls in the range of abbreviated PMR training.

Another application of EMG biofeedback is neuromuscular rehabilitation for disability related to injury or stroke.[12] This involves training increases in tension to strengthen muscles, and teaching patterns of activity in several muscle groups to enhance movement, posture, and balance. Such applications are beyond the scope of this book.

THERMAL BIOFEEDBACK (TEMP-BF). Peripheral skin temperature is related to vasodilation or constriction of the capillaries beneath the dermis: warmer temperatures reflect greater blood flow through more dilated capillaries and vice versa. Vasomotor activity is controlled by the autonomic nervous system, with sympathetic arousal producing vasoconstriction (part of the fight-or-flight response, described in Chapter One) and parasympathetic dominance leading to dilation.

In the 1960s, Elmer Green of the Menninger Clinic developed a very sensitive electronic thermal measurement and display device as part of his investigation of the apparent ability of yoga masters to exert voluntary autonomic control. Rather than the decades of meditative practice to achieve such control, Green wondered if the process could be shortened by biofeedback. In the course of their research, Elmer and his wife, Alyce Green, observed anecdotal reports of decreased migraine headache among their subjects and performed some early studies of migraine treatment by teaching temperature control.[13]

TEMP training consists of attaching a temperature sensor (thermistor) to a highly vascular area of the skin, typically a fingertip. The electronic device provides an auditory or visual signal that tracks momentary changes of small temperature fluctuations. Usually, the goal is to teach vasodilation and so, for example, a tone becomes progressively lower as temperature increases. Treatment programs for migraine include TEMP training combined with a variety of other relaxation methods in a "package" approach.[14,15] TEMP training has been employed in a similar manner in treatment programs for hypertension.[16,17] As with EMG biofeedback, the participant must be "weaned" from the machine. Instructions are given to change attention focus from the external signal to internal cues of warmth and relaxation. Session duration and number for TEMP training are similar to those of EMG, described above, and the same considerations apply.

Cognitive Methods

While physical methods require participants to perform specific bodily actions, even as subtle as dilating peripheral capillaries, cognitive methods ask only that participants think about certain aspects of their body or their external environment. The various procedures differ mainly on what their participants are instructed to ponder.

AUTOGENIC TRAINING (AT). This procedure was developed in the 1930s by Johannes Schultz, a German psychiatrist, and was brought to the attention of North American clinicians and practitioners by his student and colleague, Wolfgang Luthe, who immigrated to Canada after the Second World War. The two co-authored a six-volume compendium of their work in 1969.[18]

AT consists of instructing the person to get comfortable, in either a sitting or supine position, with eyes closed, and to listen to instructive phrases spoken by the trainer, either live or recorded. The participant is instructed to repeat the phrases silently and attend to the bodily sensations described. Further, participants are instructed to memorize the phrases and to employ them in daily home practice.

An initial phrase might be, "My right arm is heavy," repeated several times at thirty-second-intervals; then, "My left arm is heavy"; then, "Both arms are heavy." This is repeated for the legs. Other phrases concern warmth of hands and abdomen, cool forehead, slow and regular breathing, and being completely calm. Several training sessions are spent on each area before the next is added in cumulative fashion. In its initial formulation, AT employed dozens of phrases spread over months of training. But, like Jacobson's PMR, it has been modified and abbreviated for modern practice.

AT can be combined with other methods into treatment packages. For example, Blanchard employs AT with TEMP biofeedback for applications with migraine headache participants.[8]

MEDITATION. Meditation is rooted in ancient Eastern mystic traditions such as Taoism, Hinduism, and Buddhism. In a spiritual context, meditation is regarded as a means of purifying one's soul or connecting with principles of universal existence. Beginning in the "psychedelic sixties," the Maharishi Mahesh Yogi introduced "Transcendental Meditation™" (TM) to Western audiences, and copyrighted the term. He attracted a wide following, spearheaded by pop culture icons such as The Beatles, and constructed worldwide training programs. A major feature of TM is the *mantra*, a Sanskrit sound that has vibrational properties promoting transcendence into universal consciousness. A participant's individualized mantra is ceremoniously awarded by a guru after prolonged study; it has great personal significance and is to be kept secret. Although many studies reported health benefits of TM, it remains primarily a proprietary rather than a clinical research enterprise whose aim is to gain adherents to pay for courses to achieve higher and higher levels of consciousness.

Secular interest in meditation was sparked by the purported positive outcomes in physical and mental health among TM devotees. Several variations of meditation have been developed for clinical research and application. Three of the most influential programs are described below.

RELAXATION RESPONSE (RR). Herbert Benson, a cardiologist and professor at Harvard Medical School, devised a meditation procedure to evoke what he termed the "Relaxation Response" as an antidote to the fight-or-flight response triggered by stress.[19] It is a straightforward adaptation of TM, stripped of its mystic overtones.

To begin, participants are instructed to sit comfortably with eyes closed in a quiet, distraction-free environment. They are then told to relax their muscles, beginning with their feet and working upward through the body to the face. No other relaxation exercises or instructions are provided. Next, they are told to breathe through the nose, and as they exhale to say the word, "one" silently to themselves. Benson felt "one" would suffice, or any other short word or syllable the participant might prefer, rather than a secret Sanskrit mantra. Finally, participants are instructed to focus attention on their silent repetition of their word with each exhalation. If their attention wanders, they are told to return to focus on their breathing and word. Furthermore, a "passive attitude" is emphasized; the participant cannot "try" to relax, but "allow" it to happen. During the session, the trainer gives intermittent reminders, in the form of suggestions rather than imperatives, about breathing and letting go of extraneous thoughts.

The procedure usually can be learned in a single half-hour training session. Participants are instructed to practice on their own a couple times daily. Additional sessions may be used to discuss participant difficulties or observations, and to provide encouragement. Proficiency and health benefits are related to frequency and regularity of practice.

CLINICALLY STANDARDIZED MEDITATION (CSM). Another derivation of TM was developed by Patricia Carrington,[20] a researcher and teacher at Princeton University, at about the same time and for much the same reasons as Benson. In contrast to Benson, Carrington ascribes more importance to the mantra, allowing the participant to select among sixteen resonant-sounding Sanskrit words, or a word of their own choosing, that evoke a feeling of serenity. Participants are asked to sit comfortably with their eyes open, while looking at a "pleasant object" such as a potted plant. Next, they repeat their mantra aloud, then in progressively softer tones to a whisper, and then silently. Finally, they are asked to close their eyes and silently repeat their mantra at whatever pace is comfortable. In contrast to Benson, no special attention is given to breathing. If extraneous thoughts intrude, participants are told to let them "flow," but eventually return to their silent mantra. The focus of attention in CSM is thus more variable than in RR: a visual stimulus in early parts of the session; trains of thought that may arise; and the mantra.

Initial training can usually be accomplished in an hour, and participants are asked to practice at home twice daily for about twenty minutes. Carrington markets a series of audio recordings for learning CSM, teaching CSM, and modifications of CSM for specific problems such as pain or hypertension.

MINDFULNESS-BASED STRESS REDUCTION (MBSR). Jon Kabat-Zinn, a student of Zen Buddhist meditation and a researcher at the University of Massachusetts Medical School, developed the Mindfulness-Based Stress Reduction (MBSR) procedure and founded a Stress Reduction Clinic in 1979. This initially was an eight-week structured program for chronic pain participants.[21] Mindfulness approaches have since expanded to a wide variety of applications, settings, and training formats.[22]

Training begins with a didactic presentation of the concept of mindfulness: being aware in the present moment (as opposed to thinking about past or future events) in a nonjudgemental fashion (accepting an experience without evaluating it as good or bad). Like RR, MBSR asks the participant to focus on breathing, but also to connect this with sensations arising throughout the body. In the Body Scan procedure, while lying supine, the participant's attention is systematically directed to areas of the body, working up from the toes to the scalp. Participants also are asked to observe, in a nonjudgemental and accepting manner, any emotional or valanced feelings that occur in association with a particular body area, for example, pain in the lower back. In addition to the Body Scan, training is provided for other yoga-based postures, such as sitting in the lotus position. Training sessions take thirty to forty-five minutes and are available on audio recordings for home practice.

THEORIES OF RELAXATION

Relaxation theories provide conceptual frameworks that encompass the wide variety of training procedures and their effects. Most relaxation theories are reductionist, positing physiological mechanisms that underlay the experience of relaxation and its health and psychological benefits. Early theories focused on peripheral neural mechanisms while later theories propose pathways and centers of action in the brain, following technical developments in ability to monitor cortical activity. Finally, we present a theory that relies on behavioral rather than physiological observation.

Muscular Theory

Jacobson is noted for his focus on the skeletal musculature. The root of his participants' maladies lay in chronic over-activity of their motoneurons, an excess of neuromuscular excitability resulting in heightened expenditure of nervous energy. He proposed that relaxation reduces both afferent neuromuscular output and efferent proprioceptive input, based on his research showing a reduced magnitude and increased latency of spinal reflexes when a person is relaxed.

Jacobson suspected that chronic arousal affects both skeletal muscle and autonomic-mediated smooth and cardiac muscles, leading to various illnesses. He had studied with Walter B. Cannon at Harvard in the early years of the twentieth century and was familiar with the research on the "emergency reaction."[23, 24] When faced with a threatening situation, an individual (cat or human) reacts with both autonomic and skeletal muscle arousal in preparation for "fight or flight." Later research by Gellhorn and colleagues showed anatomical and functional connections between muscle proprioceptors and the posterior hypothalamus, which controlled sympathetic arousal.[25] Thus, the many symptoms that occur in gastrointestinal and cardiovascular structures that are innervated by the autonomic nervous system, such as gastric ulcer, spastic colon, hypertension, and coronary artery disease, are ameliorated by muscular relaxation. Muscular theory thus merged into autonomic theory.

Autonomic (Unitary) Theory

The role of autonomically innervated visceral structures in stress and emotional disorders, along with the mutually inhibitory relationship between the sympathetic and parasympathetic branches, provides an easily understood mechanism of relaxation. Wolpe's[6] theory of reciprocal inhibition holds that both branches of the autonomic nervous system cannot be aroused at the same time; activation of one inhibits the other. Similarly, a person cannot be both anxious (sympathetic arousal) and relaxed (parasympathetic arousal) simultaneously. While a strong threat can easily evoke the emergency response, attenuated sympathetic arousal can be inhibited by relaxation.

Benson proposed that relaxation was a "wakeful, hypometabolic, physiologic state" that could overcome chronic medical conditions resulting from prolonged stress.[19,26] Similar to Wolpe's theory, relaxation represents a shift from sympathetic arousal to parasympathetic dominance. In addition, Benson suggested that all relaxation methods have pretty much the same effect in that they embody common features. (This is discussed below in the section on Relaxation as a Response Class.) The final outcome of training, using whatever procedure, is a single phenomenon called the "relaxation response." The common-features-of-training producing a single outcome is termed a *unitary* theory of relaxation.

A problem with regarding relaxation as the generalized dominance of the parasympathetic branch is that certain disorders are characterized by overactivity in parasympathetic structures.[27] Cerebral vasodilation in migraine, bronchial constriction in asthma, and acid secretion in gastric ulcer, are some examples. If relaxation were a matter of increased parasympathetic action, these symptoms should be exacerbated by relaxation. Such is not the case. It might be more fruitful to regard relaxation as a restoration of homeostatic autonomic balance.

Cognitive/Somatic (Dualistic) Theory

As noted earlier, certain methods instruct the participant in physical activity to produce physical changes (PMR, BRT, BF) while other procedures ask the participant to sit quietly and think about things in a certain way to achieve a quiet mental state (AT, RR, CSM, MBSR). In contrast to Benson's unitary theory, some investigators have suggested that somatic methods are best used with somatic problems, and cognitive methods for cognitive problems.[28-30]

However, it is difficult to find a clear-cut dichotomy in the training methods or the disorders for which relaxation is employed. The "somatic" methods all have cognitive components, in the sense of focusing attention, following trainer instructions, and, ultimately, silent self-instructions on what to do and what to notice. And "cognitive" procedures frequently include somatic features, such as how to place one's body during practice or how to breathe. Similarly, physical problems, such as hypertension or headache, may include cognitive factors like worry or negative self-evaluations. In turn, muscle tension often is part of psychological problems like anxiety or anger.

In clinical practice, relaxation training is seldom used as the sole element in treating an individual. Relaxation usually is one of several coping skills that are trained. For example, the two case studies presented in Chapter 1 show that teaching awareness of external environmental cues that can trigger emotional upset is crucial, as is learning to recognize problematic thoughts and feelings. Further, attention to long-term goals of treatment is important. Trying to separate mind and body is a useless enterprise.

Brain-State Theory

Another opponent to unitary relaxation response theory is the view that different procedures produce different states of cortical and sub-cortical activity which, in turn, are related to specific kinds subjective experience and/or clinical outcome. Much of this discussion concerns variety in meditation practices. For example, Travis and Shear[31] differentiate three classes of meditation based on their historical traditions, types of sensory and cognitive processes employed, and differences in EEG patterns.

J. David Creswell[32] and colleagues found that an abbreviated MBSR training program had positive effects on magnetic resonance imaging (MRI) measures of brain activity related to executive function and stress hormone production, whereas a control "relaxation" procedure, based on imagery and stretching exercises, did not. David Orme-Johnson,[33] a TM© proponent, summarizes decades of research on the cortical and other physiological effects of TM, compared to other meditation and relaxation procedures. He concludes there are marked differences among methods, with TM generally producing more favorable outcomes.

Absent brain-scan technology and other sophisticated measures of physiological activity, the clinician can only speculate about what is going on in a participant's nervous system. But what is apparent is the participant's behavior.

Four-Modality Response System Theory

Rather than a reductionist account, providing explanations in terms of neurophysiology or reified psychological constructs, we propose to stay at the level of observable behavior. Emotional arousal, stress-induced activity, and relaxation can all be described as complex behavior that occurs in four response modalities or systems.[27] Table 2.1 describes each of the modal systems and each level of observation. Relaxation is a functional replacement behavior for maladaptive emotional or stressed behavior in each of these domains. Different training methods emphasize particular modes of behavior and downplay others, but relaxation is a generalized complex response across all four modalities. This taxonomy delineates all the domains in which relaxation behavior occurs and provides a framework for analyzing various training procedures and the effects they produce.

Table 2.1
Four-modality response system with examples of relaxed behavior

Behavior Modality	Function	Relaxation Examples
Motor	Manipulates physical environment	Overt: Relaxed postures Covert: Low muscle tension
Verbal	Manipulates social environment	Overt: Rating scale Covert: Silent mantra
Visceral	Maintains internal environment	Overt: Diaphragmatic breathing Covert: Slow heart rate
Observational	Generate, seek, and differentiate stimuli	Overt: Closed eyes Covert: Pleasant imagery

Structure and Function of Behavior

Behavior in each domain has both functional and structural properties. The function of behavior is of primary interest. This relates to the effects of behavior on the environment. Environment includes one's physical surroundings, like the room in which you are sitting. There is also the social environment; the people with whom one interacts are affected by one's behavior and one, in turn, is influenced by other people. In addition, there is an internal environment, the *milieu intérieur* famously described by Claude Bernard.[34] So-called states of arousal result from perturbations of the internal environment. In an example of running behavior, heart-rate and breathing change to meet increased energy requirements, and sweating and peripheral vasodilation occur to cool the body. After exercise, homeostatic processes return the body to a resting state.

Structure refers to the biological systems and anatomical structures that underlie behavior: the organs of the body and their neural connections. In turn, behavior produces changes in the body. For example, the musculoskeletal, cardiovascular, and respiratory systems allow a person to run. A regular program of running then impacts these systems. The health benefits of relaxation reflect the effect of behavior on bodily systems and structures.

Overt and Covert Behavior

Activity in each modality occurs both overtly and covertly. Overt behavior is simply that which, in principle, can be observed by another person. An outside observer can see, hear, touch, and may even smell or taste the behavior. For example, someone could see you running, or hear your footsteps and heavy breathing, or reach out and touch you as you pass by, or perhaps smell or taste the sweat that is the byproduct of running.

Covert behavior can only be observed by the individual performing that action, not by an external observer. Private behavior is that which occurs under one's skin.[35] For example, a sprinter may covertly rehearse their start before a race. An outside observer would only see a person sitting quietly with eyes closed, while the runner is seeing the lane lines converging in the distance, the feeling of getting settled into the blocks, hearing the starter say, "set," tensing muscles while rising into position, hearing the report of the starting horn, and feeling the explosion out of the blocks.

Table 2.2 shows the four-response modalities with an example of emotional and relaxed behavior at overt and covert levels in each modality. "Anxiety," "anger," or "relaxation" are complex behaviors that span all four response modes.

Motor Behavior

As the name implies, motor behavior functions to move one's body through the physical environment, as in walking, or to manipulate objects in that environment, as in grasping a tool. Structurally, it involves the skeletal muscular system and its associated neural structures in the brain, spinal cord, and peripheral nerves. Motor behavior is controlled by reflex networks and by contingencies of reinforcement in the physical and social environment, including instructions and modeling. It is also involved in other modes of behavior as described in the following sections.

Relaxed motor behavior is characterized by low levels of activity in muscle groups not required for movement or postural maintenance. As a result, publicly observable relaxed behaviors can be observed and directly measured using the Behavioral Relaxation Scale (BRS), described in Chapter 3. Covertly, muscle tension may be observed by the individual. The electromyograph, invented by Jacobson, allows overt measures of covert muscle tension, although, as Skinner noted, "the scales read by the scientist are not the same as the private events themselves" (p. 226).[36]

Relaxation does not require inactivity. Relaxed motor behavior may occur while the person engages in movement. This is the goal of training in dance and various athletic endeavors, resulting in smooth, rhythmic, and coordinated performance. Active motor relaxation in everyday life may be enhanced by training in Tai Chi[37] or the Alexander Technique[38], though further research is needed.

Anxi-us motor behavior involves the "flight" component of the fight-or flight response. Persons confronted with an anxiety-evoking situation try to

Table 2.2
Four-modality response system (4MRS) with examples of anxiety, angry and relaxed behavior at over and covert levels

Motor			Verbal			Visceral			Observational		
Anxious	*Angry*	*Relaxed*	*Anxious*	*Angry*	*Relaxed*	*Anxious*	*Angry*	*Relaxed*	*Anxious*	*Angry*	*Relaxed*
Avoid Escape Pacing	Attack Clenched jaw, fists	Relaxed postures	Reported fear, worry Reported anxiety on a scale	Reported anger, curse, threaten	Reported calm, Self-reported relaxation	Pallor, goose bumps, cold hands	Flushed face, rapid breathing	Slow breathing, warm hands	Vigilance	Glare at the enemy, Look for insults	Observe relaxed behavior
Feel tense	Feel tense	Feel calm	Self talk about fear, doom, catastrophe	Self talk about anger, unjust treatment	Self-instructions to relax, mantra, autogenic phrases	Increased heart rate, blood pressure, feel dizzy, "flight" arousal	Increased blood pressure, feel hot, "fight" arousal	Homeostasis	Attend to emotional upset; Imagine or "relive" the bad situation	Imagine ("see") the attack behavior and its effect	Attend to warmth, heaviness; imagine a calming scene

31

remove themselves from it immediately (escape) and to arrange their lives so as not to contact it again (avoidance). Phobic anxiety is classified in terms of the situations evoking escape and avoidance; for example heights, closed-in spaces, snakes, dentist offices, and so on. If escape is impossible, people become very tense and agitated, which may be seen in the form of trembling or fidgeting.

The motor components of angry behavior prepare the individual to "fight" or to damage or remove the source of upset. People may actually lash out by hitting, kicking, biting, or using a weapon on the perceived enemy. Or they may take it out on the environment, tearing up or throwing objects, or punching the wall. Even if no attack occurs, muscles associated with aggressive actions are tensed, as in making a fist. The angry person may notice covert muscle tension in certain areas, such as the jaw or shoulders.

Verbal Behavior

This mode of behavior functions to mediate social reinforcement.[39] It is the primary means by which one controls, and is controlled by, the social environment. It is acquired via principles of social learning, modeling, and differential reinforcement playing important roles. Structurally, the vocal apparatus—the lungs, larynx, pharynx, tongue, and lips, with their related neural connections and specialized brain areas—has evolved in humans in such a way so as to permit spoken language. In addition, humans have invented systems of writing and sign language. These involve motor responses in the service of verbal behavior. Receptive language requires observational behavior: listening to spoken productions; visual reading of written, signed, and gestural forms of verbal behavior; and touching (braille, finger-spelling) for blind and deaf-blind individuals. Thus, verbal behavior includes motor and observational components.

There are many verbal components to relaxation. Overt relaxed verbal behavior is characterized by public statements of calm and well-being, and by positive ratings on self-report scales. These may be taken as public announcements of private events, although social contingencies influencing such reports must be considered—people may say what they expect the listener wants to hear. Covert relaxed verbal behavior includes attending to the trainer's instructions and, later, repeating those instructions silently to oneself. One may silently repeat a mantra or statements concerning being calm and peaceful.

Additional means of communicating involve nonverbal behavior. This includes vocalizations and the prosodic features of speaking, facial expressions, gestures, and body movement and postures. These are important factors in expressing moods and emotions.[40] But systematic study of this class of behavior in the context of therapy or clinical assessment is lacking.

Overt anxious verbal behavior includes self-report of feeling afraid, such as telling another person or marking a self-report scale of anxiety. People may talk about their symptoms of anxiety, such as muscle tension or clammy hands. Fear is also communicated nonverbally, through facial expression and trembling speech delivery. Worry may be characterized as covert verbal behavior, silently telling oneself all the bad things that might happen or one's inability to deal with a fearsome situation.

Angry verbal behavior most commonly involves cursing and threatening harm, as well as self-report ("I'm mad as hell and I'm not going to take it anymore!"). The manner of speaking is obvious, with shouting and perhaps disjointed presentation. There are also characteristic facial expressions, body postures, and gestures that communicate anger. Threats and curses may be uttered covertly, as indicated by the phrase, "muttering under one's breath."

Visceral Behavior

Responses in this modality function to regulate the internal environment. Structurally, it consists of smooth and cardiac muscle and glandular systems innervated by the autonomic nervous system. It is controlled by reflex mechanisms and respondent conditioning procedures. Some responses can be affected by muscular activity, for example tensing skeletal muscles produces changes in electrodermal responses, and breathing and cardiac action are increased by physical exertion. Observational behavior also influences visceral responding: viewing a sad scene can elicit crying or an erotic scene can evoke sexual arousal.

Slow, regular breathing is a good example of overt relaxed visceral behavior. A slow, regular heartbeat can be monitored by feeling a person's pulse. Covertly, a person may be able to feel their own heartbeat, and detect peripheral vasodilation in the form of warm hands. The absence of visceral arousal, like low muscle tension, contributes to the subjective sense of calmness.

Overt visceral responses characterizing anxiety can include peripheral vasoconstriction (facial pallor or cold hands). Sweating may occur when anxious even though there is no muscular exertion (cold sweat). Piloerection (gooseflesh) sometimes happens when frightened, and borborygmus (rumbling of the gut) may be heard when anxiety disrupts digestion. In cases of extreme fright, bladder or bowel evacuation may occur. Privately, an anxious person may feel a dry mouth and slight disturbances in stomach or intestinal activity. A person prone to panic attack is usually acutely aware of visceral activity and a local disturbance, say a racing heart, can set off a cascade of other reactions.

Anger is characterized by peripheral vasodilation which may be seen as a reddened face and throbbing carotid arteries in the neck and temples; sweating often occurs. Breathing may become heavy and audible. Blood pressure typically rises, though this cannot be observed without instrumentation. Covertly, the person feels hot and may be aware of pounding heart.

Observational Behavior

The function of observational behavior is to generate, seek out and select among stimuli in one's environment. It subsumes the processes of sensation, perception, and attention. Structurally, it involves the sensory systems (visual, auditory, olfactory, gustatory, somatosensory, vestibular) including their neural connections in the periphery and brain.

Observation is necessarily an internal action, occurring within the sensory system. In some circumstances, overt motor behavior is involved to bring certain sensory receptors into contact with the environment, as in turning one's head to look at or listen to a source of stimulation, or moving one's arm and hand to touch an object or to place something in the mouth for tasting. But for definitional purposes, overt observational behavior refers to occasions where the stimulating environment is publicly available. That is, another person in that situation could observe the same events. Covert observation refers to generating or attending to private events. This includes covertly observing interoceptive stimuli, such as muscle tension or gastric motility, but also generating a covert observational stimulus for example, engaging in visual imagery—"Seeing in the absence of the thing seen" as Skinner[41] trenchantly described it. The term "earworm" has become popular, denoting covert listening to a tune no longer present in the external environment.

Relaxed overt observational behavior includes attending to the trainer's instructions or descriptions, or a biofeedback signal, or observing one's own relaxed postures. This is enhanced by a quiet environment that excludes distracting stimuli. Covertly, one can attend to the private sensations of relaxation, such as warmth and heaviness in various parts of the body. One can conjure a quiet, peaceful scene, such as water lapping on a tropical beach.

Anxious overt observational behavior is characterized by vigilance for external environmental cues that might signal the need to escape or avoid. A person who fears flying is alert to every creak or quiver of the aircraft. A person with social anxiety scans others' faces for signs of approval or disapproval. Covertly, a socially anxious person may "replay" an interaction, dissecting it for things that went wrong. As described above, an anxious person often is especially attuned to visceral events: a pounding heart feels like it's bursting; one may feel drenched in sweat; breathlessness may indicate impending loss of consciousness or death.

Angry observational behavior involves focusing on the threatening person or situation. Anything the opponent says or does is taken as a provocation. Attempts to distract an angry person are often rebuffed. Typically, an angry person is not attentive to private events, such as muscle tension or pounding heartbeat. Even pain from a wound may not be felt in the moment.

RELAXATION AS A RESPONSE CLASS

We propose that relaxation is a response class with behavior in all four modalities. A response class is comprised of elements that covary; they serve the same response function or share the effect of reinforcement or punishment. The occurrence of one behavior in the class is likely to increase the frequency of other members of the response class. This can occur within a modality (e.g., decreased muscle tension in the forehead may be associated with decreased jaw tension), and across modalities (e.g., low levels of muscle tension in the face may be related to the verbal statement, "I feel calm"). Such covariation is responsible for generalized relaxation effects of different training methods.

Common Features

There are features common to all training procedures which address the four response modalities, though in slightly different ways. Benson[19] (1975, p. 468) listed four such features: mental device; passive attitude; decreased muscle tonus; quiet environment. We consider each of these in terms of the four-modality framework.

MENTAL DEVICE. This concerns attending behavior (attention) to which the participant is directed by the trainer. In other words, the participant is directed to observe their own behavior in various modalities. In meditation, the focus is upon the mantra which the participant silently repeats (covert verbal behavior), and, in some methods, also upon breathing exhalation (overt visceral behavior). In PMR, the participant attends to the proprioceptive stimuli of muscle tension and release (covert motor behavior). For BRT, the focus is on postures (overt motor) and the proprioceptive sensations arising therefrom (covert motor), and breathing (overt visceral). AT asks the participant to observe the silent recitation of autogenic phrases (covert verbal) along with associated sensations of warmth or coolness (covert visceral) and heaviness (covert motor) in various parts of the body. Biofeedback employs overt observation of an auditory signal as well as relaxed muscle (covert motor) for EMG or warmth (covert visceral) for TEMP. MBSR also includes covert observation of breathing and on areas of the body.

PASSIVE ATTITUDE. This entails verbal instructions, which the participant may silently repeat, to avoid evaluating one's performance; to allow changes to occur and notice what happens rather than try to force an outcome, which would be counterproductive. Again, this is a directive (ply) from the trainer for the patient to engage in private observational behavior (pliance).[41] It is particularly emphasized in the meditative procedures and AT, whereas in early stages of PMR and BRT the participant is actively directed and given feedback on performance. In later stages, the emphasis shifts to more self-managed observation. In biofeedback, the signal is described in constructive rather than evaluative terms.

DECREASED MUSCLE TONUS. This refers to covert motor behavior which is the direct target of PMR, BRT, and EMG. In EMG biofeedback it occurs locally in the site trained and may generalize to other parts of the body. Muscle relaxation is presumed to occur indirectly in the meditation procedures and AT, when the participant is simply told to sit comfortably. Similarly, TEMP training may incidentally facilitate decreases in muscle tension.

QUIET ENVIRONMENT. All training procedures are conducted in quiet settings, and participants are instructed to engage in home practice at times and places free from distractions. This allows the participant to observe the "mental device" without competition for attention by extraneous stimuli. When people become proficient, they may be able to engage in mini-relaxations or take a breather in more noisy, everyday settings.

RULES FOR RELAXATION. Another feature common to all methods is providing the participant with a reason for the procedure they are about to undertake. In clinical settings, people present themselves with problems they want to resolve. It is up to the trainer to provide an explanation of the procedure and its expected benefits. Such rationales, in behavioral terms, comprise rules for undergoing training. A rule is a verbal statement of behavioral contingencies.[42,43] A rule states three terms: Antecedents—If, in certain environmental circumstances such as the training setting; Behavior—you engage in the prescribed exercises; Consequences—then you will experience relaxation and amelioration of your symptoms. Rule-governed behavior becomes an important component of self-management of stress and anxiety using relaxation in the natural environment.

Often the consequences of relaxation training are delayed or accrue only after a lengthy period of practice. An important function of rules is to bridge the temporal gap between behavior and its outcome. The trainer's rationale also enhances perception of the efficacy of the procedure by citing success obtained by others, either individual cases or group averages. In addition, the trainer can describe theoretical mechanisms—physiological or cognitive structures—that underlie the procedure and connect it with positive outcomes.

Rules are portable. Participants can incorporate them into their own verbal repertoires, allowing self-direction of their behavior in everyday settings. Participants' understanding of a procedure is inferred from their ability to repeat and follow the rules.

Another rule, usually implicit, is that the trainer's approval is contingent on the participant following instructions and reporting desired outcomes. The trainer, seen as an expert with special knowledge and skills, is a potent reinforcing agent. Trainer approval is an immediate consequence that keeps the participant on task and bridges the delay between practice and symptom change. A corollary of this is that participants' verbal behavior, their self-reports, are influenced not only by private feelings of relaxation, but by the social contingencies of the training situation as well. There is no easy control for this in a clinical setting, but the trainer should be aware of it. It points to the usefulness of multi-modal assessment. These matters will be addressed more fully in Chapter 3.

CONCLUSIONS

Relaxation training has been employed for nearly a century in the treatment of stress-related and emotional disorders. Many different methods and variations of those methods have been developed; eight are briefly described here. Procedurally, two of them require physical activity in the initial stages (PMR, BRT), and two require special equipment (EMG, TEMP). All techniques ask the participant to pay attention to some aspect of their body, differing mainly in the targets of focus, and all emphasize a passive attitude—allowing rather than forcing relaxation to occur. All methods also provide a rationale, providing an explanation to the participant on how the procedure produces relaxation and why that is important. For a few of the procedures, the basics can be learned in a session or two (RR, BRT, EMG, TEMP), though further practice is needed for proficiency. Others (PMR, AT, MBSR) have several stages that take many sessions to work through.

Most theories of relaxation are reductive, referring to events at the physiological level to account for relaxation. The skeletal-muscle system, the autonomic nervous system, and a variety of cortical and subcortical patterns of brain activity have been put forward. Instead, we propose a framework that remains at the level of observable behavior. Relaxation is regarded as a complex behavior with components across four domains: motor, verbal, visceral, and observational. Furthermore, these modes of behavior occur at both the overt level, which can, in principle, be monitored by an external observer, and the covert level, which only the behaving individual is privy to. Relaxed behavior is effective to the extent that it counteracts or replaces problematic behavior in any or all of these domains.

ENDNOTES

[1] Jacobson, E. (1929). *Progressive relaxation*. Chicago: University of Chicago Press.

[2] Jacobson, E. (1934). *You must relax*. Oxford, England: Whittlesey House.

[3] Jacobson, E. (1959). *How to relax and have your baby*. NY: McGraw-Hill.

[4] Jacobson, E. (1963). *Tension control for businessmen*. NY: McGraw-Hill.

[5] Jacobson, E. (1970). *Modern treatment of tense participants: Including the neurotic and depressed with case illustrations, follow-ups, and EMG measurements*. Springfield, IL: Charles C. Thomas, Publisher.

[6] Wolpe, J. (1958). *Psychotherapy by reciprocal inhibition*. Stanford, CA: Stanford University Press.

[7] Bernstein, D. A. & Borkovec, T. D. (1973). *Progressive relaxation Training*. Champaign, IL: Research Press.

[8] Blanchard, E. B. & Andrasik, F. (1985). *Management of chronic headaches*. New York: Pergamon.

[9] Schilling, D. J. & Poppen, R. (1983). Behavioral relaxation training and assessment. *Journal of Behavior Therapy and Experimental Psychiatry, 14*, 99–107. https://doi.org/10.1016/0005-7916(83)90027-7

[10] Budzynski, T.H., & Stoyva, J. M. (1969). An instrument for producing deep muscle relaxation by means of analog information feedback. *Journal of Applied Behavior Analysis, 2*, 231–237. https://doi.org/10.1901/jaba.1969.2-231

[11] Budzynski, T.H., Stoyva, J. M., & Adler, C.S. (1970). Feedback-induced muscle relaxation: Application to tension headache. *Journal of Behavior Therapy and Experimental Psychiatry, 1*, 205–211. https://doi.org/10.1016/0005-7916(70)90004-2

[12] Giggins, O.M., McCarthy, U., & Caufield, B. (2013). Biofeedback in rehabilitation. *Journal of Neuroengineering and Rehabilitation, 2013 10*:60. https://doi.org/10.1186/1743-0003-10-60

[13] Green, E., & Green, A. (1979). General and specific aspects of thermal biofeedback. In J.V. Basmajian (Ed.), *Biofeedback: Principles and procedures for clinicians*. Baltimore, MD: Williams & Wilkins Co.

[14]Andrasik, F. & Schwartz, M.S. (20016. Headache. In M.S. Schwartz & F. Andrasik, (Eds.), Biofeedback: A practitoner's guide, (4th ed., pp.305–355). NY: Guilford Press.

[15]Blanchard, E. B., & Andrasik, F. (1985). *Management of chronic headaches.* NY: Pergamon.

[16]Blanchard, E. B., McCoy, G. C., Musso, A., Gerardi, M.A., Pallmever, T. P., Gerardi, R. J., Cotch, P. A., Siracusa, K., & Andrasik, F. (1986). A controlled comparison of thermal biofeedback and relaxation training in the treatment of essential hypertension: I. Short-term and long-term outcome. *Behavior Therapy, 17,* 563–579. https://doi.org/10.1016/S0005-7894(86)80095-8

[17]Linden, W., & McCoy, A.V. (2016). Essential Hypertension. In M.S. Schwartz & F. Andrasik (Eds.), *Biofeedback: A Practitioner's Guide,* (4th ed., pp. 383–399). NY: Guilford Press.

[18]Schultz, J. H. & Luthe, W. (1969). *Autogenic training* (Vol. 1). NY: Grune & Stratton.

[19]Benson, H. (1975). *The relaxation response.* NY: William Morrow.

[20]Carrington, P. (1977). *Freedom in meditation.* NY. Doubleday.

[21]Kabat-Zinn, J. 1982. An out-patient program in behavioral medicine for chronic pain participants based on the practice of mindfulness meditation: Theoretical considerations and preliminary results. *General Hospital Psychiatry, 4*(1), 33–47. https://doi.org/10.1016/0163-8343(82)90026-3

[22]Williams, J.M.G., & Kabat-Zinn, J. (2013). *Mindfulness: Diverse perspectives on its meaning, origins, and applications.* NY: Routledge.

[23]Cannon, W. (1929). *Bodily changes in pain, hunger, fear, and rage.* NY: Appleton-Century-Crofts.

[24]Cannon, W. (1932). *Wisdom of the body.* NY: W.W. Norton & Company.

[25]Gellhorn, E., & Loofbourrow, G. N. (1963). Emotions and emotional disorders: A neurophysiological study. NY: Harper & Row.

[26]Wallace, R. K., Benson, H., & Wilson, A. F. (1971) A wakeful hypometabolic physiological state. *Journal of Physiology, 221,* 795–799. https://doi.org/10.1152/ajplegacy.1971.221.3.795

[27]Poppen, R. (1988). *Behavioral relaxation training and assessment* (1st ed). Thousand Oaks, CA: Sage.

[28]Davidson, R. J., & Schwartz, G. E. (1976). The psychobiology of relaxation and related states: A multi-process theory. In D. I. Mostofsky (Ed.), *Behavior control and modification of physiological activity* (pp. 399–442). Englewood Cliffs, NJ: Prentice Hall.

[29]Lehrer, P.M. (1996). Varieties of relaxation methods and their unique effects. *International Journal of Stress Management,3*(1), 1–15. https://doi.org/10.1007/BF01857884

[30]Lehrer, P. M., Woolfolk, R. L., Rooney, A. J., McCann, B., & Carrington, P. (1983). Progressive relaxation and meditation: A study of psychophysiological and therapeutic differences between two techniques. *Behavior Research and Therapy, 21,* 651–662. https://doi.org/10.1016/0005-7967(83)90083-9

[31]Travis, F., & Shear, J. (2010). Focused attention, open monitoring and automatic self-transcending: Categories to organize meditations from Vedic, Buddhist and Chinese traditions. *Consciousness and Cognition, 19* (4), 1110–1118. https://doi.org/10.1016/j.concog.2010.01.007

[32]Creswell, J. D., Taren, A. A., Lindsay, E. K., Greco, C. M., Gianaros, P. J., Fairgrieve, A. Marsland, A. L., Brown, K. W., Way, B. W., Rosen, R. K., & Ferris, J. L (2016). Alterations in resting-state functional connectivity link mindfulness meditation with reduced interleukin-6: A randomized controlled trial. *Biological Psychiatry, 80* (1), 53–61. https://doi.org/10.1016/j.biopsych.2016.01.008

[33]http://www.truthabouttm.org/truth/Home/AboutDavidOrme-Johnson/RecentPublica- tions/index.cfm

[34]Gross, C. G. (1998). Claude Bernard and the constancy of the internal environment. *Neuroscientist, 4*, 380–385. https://doi.org/10.1177/107385849800400520

[35]Skinner, B. F. (1953). *Science and human behavior.* NY: MacMillan

[36]Skinner, B. F. (1969). *Contingencies of reinforcement. A theoretical account.* NY: Appleton-Century-Crofts.

[37]Wu, J. & Poppen, R. (1996). *Physiological and psychological effects of Tai Chi practice.* Association for Applied Psychophysiology and Biofeedback, Albuquerque, NM.

[38]Brennan, R. (1996). *The Alexander technique manual.* Boston: Journey Editions.

[39]Skinner, B. F. (1957). *Verbal behavior.* Acton, MA: Copley Publishing Group.

[40]Knapp, M. L., Hall, J. A., & Horgan, T. G. (2014). *Nonverbal communication in human interaction.* (8th Ed.). Boston: Wadsworth.

[41]Skinner, B. F. (1974). *About behaviorism.* NY: Knopf.

[42]Poppen, R. (1989). Some clinical implications of rule-governed behavior. In S. C. Hayes (Ed.) *Rule-governed behavior: Cognitions, contingencies, and instructional control* (pp. 325–357). NY: Plenum.

Supplement
Behavior Analyst Certification Board 5th Edition Task List

A. Philosophical Underpinnings

A-1   Identify the goals of behavior analysis as a science (i.e., description, prediction, control).

A-2   Explain the philosophical assumptions underlying the science of behavior analysis (e.g., selectionism, determinism, empiricism, parsimony, pragmatism).

A-3   Describe and explain behavior from the perspective of radical behaviorism.

A-4   Distinguish among behaviorism, the experimental analysis of behavior, applied behavior analysis, and professional practice guided by the science of behavior analysis.

B-3   Define and provide examples of respondent and operant conditioning.

B. Concepts and Principles

B-1   Define and provide examples of behavior, response, and response class.

G. Behavior-Change Procedures

G-1   Use positive and negative reinforcement procedures to strengthen behavior.

G-14   Use reinforcement procedures to weaken behavior (e.g., DRA, FCT, DRO, DRL, NCR).

G-10   Teach simple and conditional discriminations.

G-6   Use instructions and rules.

G-20   Use self-management strategies.

F. Behavior Assessment

F-1   Review records and available data (e.g., educational, medical, historical) at the outset of the case.

Chapter 3

Assessment of Relaxation

Behavioral assessment is the general term that describes the process by which target behaviors are identified and defined, concurrent with determination of the maintaining contingencies. This functional analysis is the first step in deciding whether relaxation would be a more adaptive response to the situation than whatever the person is doing that has brought them in for treatment. The decision should be a joint one with the participant (or by responsible care-givers for persons with severe limitations), in which the treatment methods and goals are spelled out. The next step involves assessment of both treatment (relaxation training and related procedures) and the target behaviors. We maintain that it is essential to measure the degree to which the participant learns relaxation skills, along with measurement of treatment outcomes, to be sure of the relationship between the two. The insistence on assessment of the fidelity the treatment[1-6] (implementation and processes outcomes) and treatment outcome measures buttresses the claim of "evidence-based treatment," even at the level of individual cases in clinical settings.

This chapter first examines function-based assessment as the basis for implementing relaxation training. Next, we emphasize the importance of assessing treatment. A number of self-report measures of relaxation are described. The main focus of the chapter is on a direct-observation measure of relaxation, the Behavioral Relaxation Scale (BRS). Finally, relationships among the various measures are discussed.

FUNCTION-BASED ASSESSMENT AND RELAXATION

The role and importance of a functional approach to behavioral assessment has grown in the last forty years. Skinner[7] described functional analysis as the extent of experimental control over a behavior as a function of consequent events. Clinical application of function-based assessment was described by Ferster[8] and elaborated on by Kanfer and Saslow[9] who described it as a process where "...the eventual therapeutic methods can be directly related to the information obtained in the continuing assessment of the participant's current behaviors and controlling stimuli"(p. 533). Activities and processes aimed at describing potential controlling variables have been referred to as *functional assessment*, whereas demonstration of the controlling effect of these environmental events is the realm of *functional analysis*.[10]

An explicit characteristic of behavioral assessment is identifying meaningful (adaptive) replacement behaviors that ideally serve the same response function and could compete with the occurrence of undesired behavior. These adaptive behaviors enable the individual to gain access to more environments and make contact with more reinforcing events. Relaxation, as a complex class of behavior, is such an example.

Function-based assessment involves either descriptive (correlational) or experimental analysis and strives to identify controlling environment-behavior relations. As noted in Chapter 1 with Larry (and in many cases in later chapters), function-based assessment plays an integral role in the selection of relaxation as an alternative response.

Indirect measurement takes place in the clinical interview with the participant, direct-care staff, or other caregivers to obtain the participant's history. The goal is to establish a behavioral diagnosis that reveals the current modes of responding that are problematic and the conditions under which they occur. Functional analysis, widely used in research with individuals with intellectual disabilities and autism spectrum disorder,[11] is followed by replacement behavior selection and intervention. Relaxation is a socially valid replacement behavior[12] and should be considered, especially when the goal is self-management. Reinforcing consequences for the problematic behaviors, such as attention from others, monetary compensation, medication, and escape/avoidance of tasks and responsibilities, need to be examined. The participant's history may reveal the antecedents of their behavior and physical symptoms—the social and physical environments that increase the likelihood of problematic behavior. These antecedent events provide clues to the situations in which relaxation will be most useful.

As discussed in Chapter 2, problem behaviors occur in any and all of the four modalities of responding. Complex emotional, painful, and stress-related behaviors are costly and ineffective ways of coping with life's demands. Values clarification, using the *bull's eye task*, is a helpful method to employ shortly after the initial intake and interview.[13] Completion of the bull's eye task allows a review of the costs and discomforts the participant is experiencing and enhances the potential reinforcing value of relaxation as an alternative response that allows greater ability to live a more meaningful life. Brief motivational interviewing, focusing on the benefits of behavior change (relaxation), is a verbally-mediated motivating operation related to the benefits of treatment. This verbal interaction between the therapist and participant regarding the benefits of behavior change begins to establish rule-governed behavior[14] through the therapist directly stating the rule (a ply)[15] or shaping the verbal behavior of the participant to abstract and state the rule: In this case, "When I am stressed, if I relax I will feel better and I can get through the day." Working with the participant to pinpoint eliciting and evoking stimuli related to the problem behavior allows the therapist to develop procedures for decreasing or removing such antecedents, as well as teaching relaxation skills to use when such situations arise.

ASSESSMENT OF TRAINING

The paradigm for teaching a skill involves the following steps:

1. Instruction;
2. Assess student performance;
3. Reinforce progress;
4. Remediate errors;
5. Move to next stage of training.

Steps 3, 4, and 5 all depend on Step 2, assessment. This much is a truism in any educational enterprise and hardly bears repeating. However, teachers of relaxation routinely neglect measurement of their pupils' performance.

One reason for this omission may be the presumption that relaxation training, by definition, produces relaxation. The clinician provides treatment (e.g., PMR), and the participant experiences an outcome (e.g., reported reduction in headaches). This is the critical relationship, and the clinician need not be concerned about what may be happening in between training and outcome. Similarly, a researcher may compare one treatment (e.g., PMR) to another (e.g., attention-placebo), with the outcome again being headache reduction. Or, the researcher may compare a combination treatment (e.g., PMR + cognitive therapy) to each of the components individually. By careful control of extraneous variables, it is possible to demonstrate that the outcome is statistically more probable with one intervention compared to another.

The researcher's concern with probabilities raises a critical point. Relationships between treatments and outcomes are never black or white. Not all persons given PMR improve; not all persons given attention-placebo fail to improve. Clinicians and researchers are constantly seeking to improve their odds for success, and looking at the direct effects of training provides one means of doing so. To use a medical analogy, in cases where a participant fails to improve, is it is because the participant failed to take the pills or because the medication did not work? Only by assessing the intermediate stage, the level of medication in the participant's system, can answers be obtained and treatment odds improved. The crucial relationship is not between the prescription of medication and outcome, but rather between biochemical action and outcome. Similarly, providing relaxation training is not the same thing as the participant actually learning a skill and employing it in daily living. Assessing the participant's proficiency in relaxation makes it possible to determine a dose-response relationship, which is a very powerful way of assessing treatment effectiveness.

Treatment integrity is an important issue: to what degree has the intervention been delivered "as advertised?"[1-6] To use the medical analogy, are the pills ingested in the prescribed manner? It is important, especially in research settings, that interventions are carried out as specified. However, providing treatment is not the same as the participant learning a skill. Determining the relationship between relaxation treatment and outcome requires not only that the therapist administer training in the prescribed manner, but also that the participant demonstrates that relaxation has been learned. In addition, assessment of relaxation allows the trainer to provide guidance, correction, and reinforcement—in short, to teach rather than merely instruct.

Another problem with looking at outcome as the only dependent measure is that often it is based on participant self-report of subjective symptoms. The difficulties with this measure are discussed in a later section. Suffice it to say here that many variables in addition to the intervention can influence self-report. To strengthen the claim of treatment effectiveness, it is important to measure what happens to participants during training while they are available for objective observation. The degree of relaxation achieved in training is presumed to be a precursor of relaxation in the natural environment, which is one of the variables affecting self-report of symptoms. Thus, the assessment of relaxation gives the clinician and researcher one more handle by which to grasp the relationship between treatment and outcome.

SELF-REPORT MEASURES OF RELAXATION

A relatively easy way for clinicians or researchers to assess if the participant is learning relaxation is to ask them how they feel. The widespread notion of relaxation as an internal state leads to a reliance on the participant as the primary observer of that state. Consequently, the trainer may gauge the participant's progress by their answer to the question, "How did that go?" or "How do you feel?" Comments by the participant such as, "I feel like I am melted in the chair" or "I just can't seem to let myself go" are taken as primary data on the subjective state of relaxation. More rigorous attempts to quantify relaxation have led to a variety of rating scales.

THE SUD SCALE   The Subjective Unit of Distress Scale (SUDS) asks for a rating of anxiety or arousal from 0 to 100.[16] Although couched in terms of arousal, low SUDS ratings may be regarded as measures of calmness or relaxation.

TENSION SELF-RATING SCALE   Schilling and Poppen[17] employed a 7-point tension scale, with associated descriptors of relaxation and arousal (e.g., 1 = "Feeling deeply and completely relaxed throughout my entire body"; 4 = "Feeling relaxed as in my normal resting state"; 7 = "Feeling extremely tense and upset throughout my entire body." See Appendix A). This has been employed in many clinical and research settings.

VISUAL ANALOG SCALE   Other investigators have employed an analog scale.[18-20] This provides the participant with a 10-cm horizontal line on a piece of paper, with one end labeled *very tense* and the other end labeled *very relaxed*. The person simply makes a mark on the line. This is then converted to a percentage by measuring the distance from one end of the line to the mark and dividing by ten.

RELAXATION INVENTORY (RI)   The Relaxation Inventory (RI) is a 45-item questionnaire on which respondents endorse items that describe feelings.[21,22] Three subscales have been derived through factor analysis: Physiological Tension, Cognitive Tension, and Physical Assessment. Appropriate changes in subscale and total scores were obtained following PMR training, "imaginal" relaxation (in which participants were instructed to imagine themselves engaging in the relaxation exercises), and tension induction.

Hites and Lundervold[23] examined the extent to which self-reported change in physical tension and cognitive arousal were related to performance of relaxed behaviors on the BRS. These researchers were not able to replicate the construct validity of the Relaxation Inventory (RI)[21,22] when direct observation of relaxed behavior was the criterion. The three RI subscales (Physical Tension, Cognitive Tension, and Physical Assessment) were found to be significantly intercorrelated.

SMITH STATES OF RELAXATION INVENTORY (SSRI)   Smith[24] suggested that relaxation may not be fully understood without understanding the participant's report of the extent and process of relaxation. Based on the revised

Relaxation Wordlist, an 82-item inventory on which respondents rate the extent to which each word describes their relaxation experience, Smith[25,26] developed the concept of a relaxation state (R-State), to provide a universal lexicon by which to describe relaxation effects. R-States are "psychological states of mind associated with practicing relaxation and mastering the act of sustaining passive simple focus" (p. 5).[25] Initial results from nearly one thousand practitioners of various types of relaxation (e.g., PMR, Autogenic Training, Lamaze, meditation) were factor analyzed, yielding five to fourteen factors depending on the decision criteria. He then added a fifteenth factor, described as a meta-state of "awareness."[25] Based on the concept of R-States, he developed the Smith States of Relaxation Inventory (SSRI).[26] This instrument does not measure the degree of relaxation, but rather reflects various categories of self-reported sensation, emotion, and motor activity related to relaxation. Smith[25] further proposed that the meta-state "awareness" was a proxy for mindfulness. Growing ever grander, Smith[27] presented a procedure-specific effect theory of relaxation training and R-States.

Several quasi-experimental retrospective studies conducted by Smith and his students comparing the R-States of different relaxation groups have produced equivocal results.[25] Similarly, Hites and Lundervold[23] found that the R-State awareness was not related to performance of relaxed behavior. Nor was the construct validity of the SSRI established when direct observation of relaxed behavior was the criterion measure. Finally, only one prospective experimental study of relaxation training and R-States has been conducted.[28] The results of Hobbs[28] contradicts Smith's specific procedure-specific outcome theory of relaxation. Hobbs also reported ceiling effects for the SSRI due to the limited range of possible scores. While assessment of private events related to relaxation is important, further research and development of instruments is needed.

STATES OF AROUSAL AND RELAXATION (STAR) SCALE. A different approach to the assessment of the effects of relaxation was undertaken by Lundervold and colleagues. As discussed earlier, Smith[25,26] suggested that relaxation resulted in a meta-state of awareness or mindfulness; unfortunately, his measurement of mindfulness was based on only one item. Roemer[29] also suggested that relaxation produced mindfulness and used PMR exercises as part of an acceptance-based treatment package for generalized anxiety. The results of Hobbs[28] indicated that individuals trained in relaxation using BRT procedures reported increased mindfulness based on the Five Facets of Mindfulness questionnaire, which has been shown to be a valid measure of the construct.[30]

Building on the work of Hobbs, Lundervold and colleagues[31,32] developed the States of Arousal and Relaxation Scale (STAR; see Appendix B). The STAR assesses five domains: (a) revived; (b) detached; (c) cognitive arousal; (d) mindfulness; and (e) physical relaxation. In the first study of 31 participants, the STAR was found to have good stability (test-retest reliability: $r = .71$, $p = .0001$) over a two week period, and was positively and significantly associated with the Behavioral Relaxation Scale ($r = .45$, $p = .01$), a direct observation measure of relaxed behavior. Internal consistency reliability of the STAR was excellent (adjusted alpha $r = .94$). Scores on the mindfulness subscale were orthogonal to the other dimensions of the STAR, lending indirect support to the conclusion that relaxation results in self-reported mindfulness.

In a second study, a similarly sized sample was assessed using the same procedures; however, the Observe subscale of the Five Facets of Mindfulness,[30] and the Toronto Mindfulness Scale[33] were used to further examine the construct validity of the STAR with respect to mindfulness. Results supported the interpretation that the STAR measures mindfulness. Further research examining the STAR's sensitivity to change subsequent to relaxation training is needed.

Limitations of Self-Report

While it is useful to include self-reports of internal events when working with verbal participants, clinicians would do well to recognize the limitations of such behavior. The first limitation is what B.F. Skinner called "the problem of privacy."[14] Stated simply, this problem is that people have difficulty discriminating and labeling internal stimuli because they lack corrective feedback from their environment. Little Johnny learns not to call kitty "doggie," or to call the mailman "Daddy" when his mother observes the error and provides corrective consequences. But such accurate correction is not forthcoming in learning about internal events. We eventually arrive at a crude consensus about private stimuli through a slow process of metaphor (e.g., "I feel like a truck ran me over") and public accompaniments (e.g., "You seem down in the mouth"). But we never achieve the accuracy in discriminating private events that we do when people around us have direct access to, and can provide feedback on, what we are speaking about.

Another limitation of self-report is that it is so reactive to social contingencies, often to a greater extent than to internal stimuli. It is well documented that people often report feeling more relaxed after receiving some treatment that they are told is effective, even though no change has taken place in motor or visceral modalities.[34-38] Conversely, people may report no change in feelings, even though muscle tension has actually decreased, when the procedure is labeled "physiological assessment" rather than "relaxation training."[39] Part of what is termed a "placebo effect" is this change in verbal behavior in response to therapist instructions and approval.

Self-Report of Symptoms

Symptom reports are a primary dependent variable in most therapy and research endeavors involving relaxation. In some instances such as hypertension, spasmodic torticollis, and Raynaud's disease, the symptom can be measured objectively. But in many instances such as headache and other types of pain, or anxiety or other emotions, the therapist must depend on the participant's report. This report may be systematically solicited, as in a "headache diary,"[40] or more informally gathered (e.g., "Well, how's it going this week?"). Of particular concern are the social contingencies that serve to maintain such reports. For example, Fordyce[41] documented the influence of social contingencies on verbal reports of both subjective pain and overt pain behaviors.

This is not to deny that self-reports are useful and often essential measures of both relaxation states and symptom levels. But the clinician and researcher should be aware of the factors that influence self-report, and to employ more objective measures when available.

THE BEHAVIORAL RELAXATION SCALE (BRS)

Measurement of relaxation, as described in the preceding sections, usually is based on the premise that relaxation is an internal state and self-report has been used primarily to measure this covert behavior. The basic premise of the BRS is that a relaxed person engages in overt motor behavior that is characteristic of relaxation. (See Appendix C). It is possible for an external observer to take note of these behaviors and to judge how relaxed the participant is. At this point, the concern is only with relaxation in the training situation. In later sections, the issue of relaxation assessment outside the training environment is addressed. Also, the BRS is primarily a measure of the motor behavior aspects of relaxation. Description of a more complete multimodal assessment procedure concludes this chapter.

A Brief History of the BRS

As one reads the classic work of Edmund Jacobson, one is struck by the descriptive detail of what he observed in his participants.[42] His text is accompanied by many photographs showing what the outcome of training should look like. Similarly, other investigators have presented phenomenological descriptions of what transpires as a person becomes relaxed, along with hints on how to assess it. Wolpe[16,43] and Bernstein et al.[44] have been particularly helpful in this respect. The contributions of Arnold Lazarus, who instructed the second author in the arcane skill of PMR training, also should be acknowledged. After many years of teaching relaxation, as well as teaching students to teach relaxation, and those students going to work with participants and teach their own students, some "rules of thumb" for assessing relaxation have been gleaned.

Don Schilling was the first to apply these rules of thumb in a systematic fashion when he undertook relaxation training with "pre-delinquent" boys. PMR training had resulted in boys who were good at the "tensing" part but poor at "releasing." Showing some creative behavior analytic skills, Schilling decided to teach the boys to "look relaxed." Sure enough, the children not only could look relaxed, they reported that they felt relaxed and exhibited a calm demeanor after each training session. All that remained was to work out a specific list of behaviors and to formally test the reliability of observation of these behaviors and their relation to other measures. That list became the BRS.

Ten Relaxed Behaviors

The BRS consists of a description of ten postures and activities characteristic of a fully relaxed person whose body is supported by a reclining chair or similar device. First, these behaviors are described in words and photographs. Next, a method for systematically observing them is presented. Each behavior consists of an overt posture or activity of a specific region of the body. To enhance discrimination, both relaxed behaviors and some commonly occurring unrelaxed behaviors are presented for each item.

1. *Head*

RELAXED. The head is motionless and supported by the recliner, with the nose in the midline of the body. Body midline usually can be determined by clothing features such as shirt buttons or apex of V neckline. Part of the nostrils and the underside of the chin is visible (see Photo 3.1A).

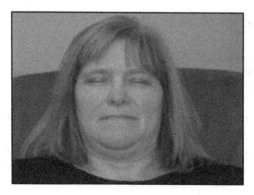

Photo 3.1A

UNRELAXED. Any of the following: (a) movement of the head; (b) head turned from body midline with the entire nose beyond midline (Photo 3.1B); (c) head tilted downward with the nostrils and underside of the chin not visible (Photo 3.1B); (d) head unsupported by the recliner; (e) head tilted upward with the underside of the chin visible (Photo 3.1C).

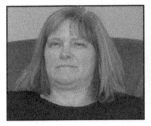 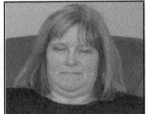 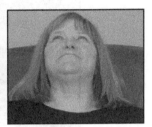

Photos 3.1A, 3.1B, and 3.1C

2. *Eyes*

RELAXED. The eyelids are lightly closed with a smooth appearance, and no motion of the eyes beneath the eyelids (see Photo 3.2A).

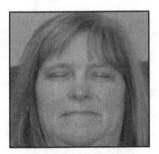

Photo 3.2A

UNRELAXED. Any of the following: (a) eyes open; (b) eyelids closed but wrinkled or fluttering (Photo 3.2B, C); (c) eyes moving under the eyelids.

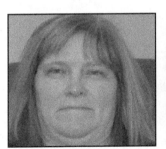 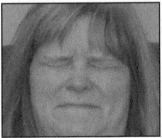

Photo 3.2B and 3.2C

3. *Mouth*

RELAXED. The lips are parted at the center of the mouth from ¼ inch to 1 inch (7–25 mm) with the front teeth also slightly parted (see Photo 3.3A).

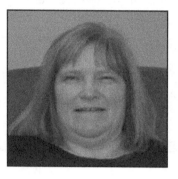

Photo 3.3A

UNRELAXED. Any of the following: (a) teeth in occlusion (Photo 3.3B); (b) lips closed (Photo 3.3C); (c) mouth open greater than 1 inch (25 mm) (in most cases, the corners of the mouth will separate when the mouth is open beyond criterion (Photo 3.3D); (d) tongue motion (e.g., licking lips).

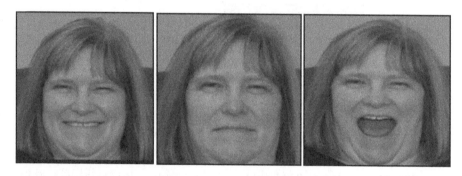

Photos 3.3B, C, and D

4. *Throat*

   RELAXED. There is an absence of motion (see Photo 3.4).

   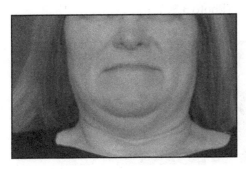
   Photo 3.4

   UNRELAXED. There is any type of movement in the throat and neck (e.g., swallowing or other larynx action, or twitches in the neck muscles).

5. *Shoulders*

   RELAXED. Both shoulders appear rounded and transect the same horizontal plane. They rest against the recliner with no motion other than respiration (see Photo 3.5A).

   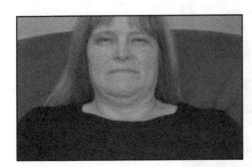
   Photo 3.5A

UNRELAXED. Any of the following: (a) movement of the shoulders; (b) shoulders on a diagonal plane (Photo 3.5B); (c) shoulders are raised or lowered so as not to appear rounded (Photo 3.5C).

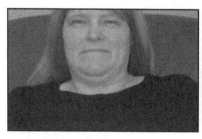
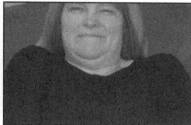

Photos 3.5B and C

6. *Body*

RELAXED. The torso, hips, and legs are symmetrical around midline, resting against the chair, with no movement (see Photo 3.6A).

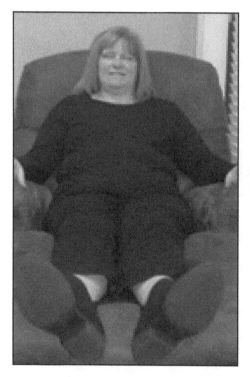

Photos 3.6A

UNRELAXED. Any of the following: (a) movement of the torso other than respiration; (b) twisting of torso, hips, or legs out of midline (Photo 3.6B); (c) any movement of the hips, legs, or arms that does not result in movement of feet or hands (these are scored separately); (d) any part of the back, buttocks, or legs not supported by the recliner.

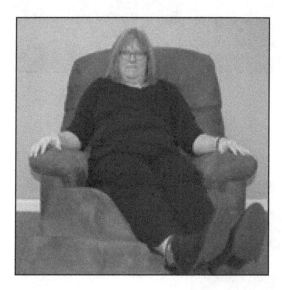

Photo 3.6B

7. Hands

RELAXED. Both hands are resting on the armrest of the chair or on the lap with palms down and the finger curled in a claw-like fashion. The fingers are sufficiently curled if a pencil can pass freely beneath the highest point of the arc other than the thumb (see Photo 3.7A).

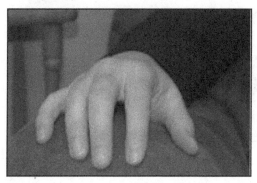

Photo 3.7A

UNRELAXED. Any of the following: (a) hands gripping the armrest (Photo 3.7B); (b) fingers extended and straight (Photo 3.7C); (c) fingers curled so that nails touch the surface of the armrest (Photo 3.7D); (d) fingers intertwined; (e) movement of the hands.

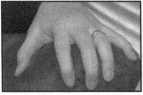 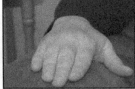 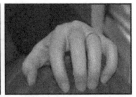

Photos 3.7B, C, and D

8. *Feet*

   RELAXED. The feet are pointed away from each other in a V at an angle between 60 and 90 degrees (see Photo 3.8A).

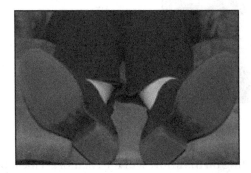

Photo 3.8A

UNRELAXED. Any of the following: (a) movement of the feet; (b) feet pointing vertically or at an angle less than 60° (Photo 3.8B); (c) feet pointing out at an angle greater than 90° (Photo 3.8C); (d) feet crossed at the ankles (Photo 3.8D); (e) one heel placed more than 1 inch (25 mm) ahead or behind the other.

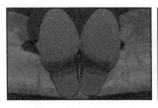 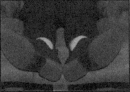 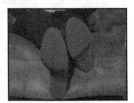

Photos 3.8B, C, and D

9. *Quiet*

   RELAXED. There are no vocalizations or loud respiratory sounds.

   UNRELAXED. Any type of verbalization or vocalization (e.g., talking, sighing, grunting, snoring, gasping, coughing).

10. *Breathing*

    RELAXED. The breath frequency is less than that observed during baseline, with no breathing interruptions. One breath equals one complete inhale-exhale cycle. A breath is counted if any part of the inhale occurs on the cue starting the observation interval and any part of the exhale occurs on the cue ending the observations interval (see how to score breathing in the section titled "Scoring the BRS").

    UNRELAXED. Any of the following: (a) breathing frequency is equal to or greater than that during baseline; (b) any irregularity that interrupts the regular rhythm of breathing (e.g., coughing, laughing, yawning, sneezing).

All relaxed behaviors are shown together in Photo 3.9. The participant can be scanned from head to feet on a systematic basis to measure relaxation, as presented in the next section.

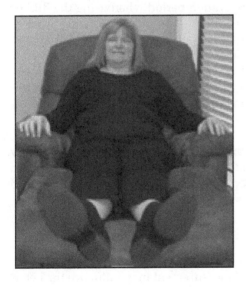

Photo 3.9

Using the BRS

One of the main uses of the BRS is to assess the degree of relaxation attained by a person participating in a relaxation training procedure. As Chapter 4 describes, the BRS is an integral part of the Behavioral Relaxation Training (BRT) procedure. And we discuss use of the BRS with other procedures later in this chapter. However, the BRS is useful by itself as a dependent measure for any relaxation training procedure chosen by the trainer. In its standard form, the BRS requires that the training be carried out with the participant seated in a reclining chair or similar device. Modifications for use with the participant seated in a straight-back chair are presented later.

Duration of the Observation Period

The BRS requires an observation period, usually at the conclusion of a relaxation training session. It may also be employed at the beginning of a session as a baseline measure of performance. The duration of the observation period must be several minutes. We have employed durations of three, five, and ten minutes. In general, the longer the period, the more representative sample of relaxed behavior will be obtained. But considerations of time constraints and participant characteristics are important and should be evaluated for each application. Five minutes is sufficient for most purposes.

Research on duration of the observation period when using the BRS has been conducted. Lundervold and Dunlap[45] examined BRS scores from ten adults. Correlation analyses of BRS scores for one, two, three, and five 60-second observation periods were conducted. All alternate durations of the BRS observation period were robustly associated with the long duration (five minute) BRS score ($r \geq 0.80$, $p = 0.005$). Alternate forms of BRS observation periods provide more flexibility in applied situations without loss of representative samples of behavior.

Each minute of the observation period is divided into three intervals: a 30-second interval to observe breathing rate, a 15-second interval to observe the other nine items on the BRS, and a 15-second interval to record the observations on the BRS Score Sheet. Copies of the BRS Score Sheet should be made for the trainer to use in assessing relaxation.

Reactivity

Any behavioral observation procedure may be reactive if the person is aware of the observation; that is, the act of measurement may influence the behavior being measured, resulting in inaccurate assessment. We have found two major areas of reactivity in employing the BRS that the user should be aware of and take steps to reduce. The two reactive features of the BRS are the discriminability of the observation period and concern over "being watched."

Discriminability of the Observation Period

It is desirable to measure relaxation in the absence of other interactions with the participant. Observation typically is carried out in silence, which may provide a cue to the participant about a change in conditions; that is, if relaxation training has employed some sort of signal or instruction administered to the participant (e.g., BIOF, PMR) and this presentation suddenly ends, then the participant may be alerted that the session is about to end. This could disrupt relaxation. We have employed instructions and an adaptation period in BRT research and practice to minimize reactivity. In research settings, we regularly employ a five-minute adaptation period in which the participant is instructed that "We are going to be taking some notes. Just relax on your own for the next few minutes." During the adaptation period, the observer may review the recording sheet while periodically looking up and toward the participant. This pre-observation interval also allows the observer to subtlety observe the participant's breathing behavior and identify the most salient component of that behavior prior to the start of the formal observation. These actions are very similar to those that occur during the BRS observation and decrease reactivity. In clinical practice the same procedure is used but the adaptation period is much shorter, usually two minutes.

At the conclusion of training we typically instruct participants to "relax on your own for the next few minutes" while we assess the effectiveness of training. This is sufficient for most people. It also is possible to incorporate an observation period within the training session or to continue to administer treatment until the end of the session so that there are no changes to alert the participant.

Concern About Being Watched

This is another reactive aspect of BRS observation. Although not widespread, it is most evident in initial stages of training when baseline measures are being collected. It is at this time when the procedures are the most unfamiliar to the participant and also the time when the participant is most likely to have their eyes open, watching the trainer watch them. This can be particularly unnerving. "Eyes closed" is one of the items on the BRS, and instructions to the participant to close their eyes would be a confound in the baseline period of a research project. In clinical practice it is more likely that the participant will close their eyes when instructed to relax in the baseline condition; it does no harm if the participant closes their eyes or is instructed to do so.

This merely inflates the baseline relaxation score by ten percent and can be noted accordingly. In addition, the participant should be instructed in the rationale given at the start of their training procedure that it is necessary to measure the effects of the training and that, therefore, they will be observed periodically. The emphasis should be that it is the training procedure that is being measured, rather than how well the participant is performing, to avoid undue performance pressure. Examples of such instructions are given in a later section.

Generally, the participant becomes more at ease as training progresses and observation is accepted as part of the procedure. Where facilities permit, it may be possible to observe the participant through a one-way window or to use a video camera to view or record an observation period. Not seeing the observer may put the participant more at ease. When this is done, ethical practice requires that the person be informed that observation is taking place. In all cases, either clinical or research, every effort should be made to establish good rapport between the trainer and participant and to assure the latter that confidentiality always is maintained.

Positioning the Observer

The observer should place themselves in a position to obtain a full and unobstructed view of the participant. Because symmetry around midline is an important aspect of several items on the BRS, the observer should not be seated completely to one side of the participant. Nor should the observer sit directly at the foot of the recliner; if the participant's feet are elevated, they may block the observer's view of breathing, body, or hands; or if the participant is wearing a skirt, then such a position may be inappropriate. We have found that placing the observer to one side at the foot of the recliner, at the "5 o'clock" or "7 o'clock" position, provides a good view of symmetry and all behaviors listed on the BRS. The observer should be seated about one to one-and-a-half meters from the participant. The room should be lighted well enough to permit observation of small movements, but the light should not be so bright as to disrupt relaxation, nor should the light be directed in the participant's eyes. All these considerations are especially important in the placement of a video camera or a one-way window, both of which tend to restrict observation.

Timing Device

The observer requires a timing device to divide each minute of the observation period into appropriate scoring intervals. One option is to use an electronic stopwatch attached to a clipboard holding the BRS Recording Form.

When using a stopwatch, the observer must be careful not to avert their eyes from the participant and perhaps miss the occurrence of unrelaxed behavior. Alternatively, a large clock with a sweep second hand or digital readout of seconds may be placed just behind the participant, allowing the observer to view the clock as he or she scans the participant. Another method is to put time cues on a digital player/recording device, which then can be played by the observer and heard unobtrusively through a small ear bud.

Observational Procedure

Before starting the observation period, the observer should write the participant's name or identification code on the BRS Recording Form (Appendix C). The date, time, session number, and other relevant training data should also be written down. The participant's baseline breathing rate, determined from baseline sessions, should be written in the box at the top of the BRS form. The method used to determine a person's baseline breathing rate is described in a later section. Direct observation of relaxed behavior employs continuous and discontinuous measurement systems and use of interval observation. Continuous recording of breathing is used within each interval. Whole-interval recording is used with the remaining nine behaviors. In this case, the relaxed behavior must occur for the entire interval to be scored as an occurrence. Relaxed behavior is scored as a plus (+) for the specified interval of time; unrelaxed behavior is scored as a minus (–).

The first behavior observed and scored in each interval is Breathing. With the onset of each minute of the observation period, the observer determines whether or not the participant is inhaling. If so, then an inhale-exhale cycle has commenced; if not, then the observer waits until the next inhale before beginning the count. Each inhale-exhale cycle is counted as one breath. When the timing device indicates that thirty seconds have elapsed, the observer stops counting breaths. If the participant is exhaling at the end of the breathing observation interval, then the cycle is counted as a complete breathing. If the participant is inhaling at the end of the interval, then the breath is not counted. The observer records the number of breaths in the box at the top of each column of the BRS Score Sheet in the row marked Breathing. If an interruption to breathing occurs (see description of Unrelaxed Breathing in previous section) the interval is spoiled and the observer marks an "S" the in box.

For the fifteen seconds following observation of Breathing, the observer scans the participant for any unrelaxed behavior among the other nine items listed on the BRS. If an unrelaxed behavior is observed, the observer may silently repeat the one-word label for that behavior to aid recall until the end of the interval. If recall is a problem, then the observer may immediately draw a slash (/) through the minus sign in the appropriate column of the

BRS Score Sheet in the row of the particular item noted. This should be done quickly so as not to miss other occurrences of unrelaxed behavior.

For the final fifteen seconds of each minute, the observer slashes the minus signs in the appropriate rows for any unrelaxed behavior observed in the preceding interval. If no unrelaxed behaviors were noted, then the appropriate plus signs are marked. The breathing rate written in the small box at the top of each column is compared to the baseline breathing rate. If the rate is less than baseline, then the plus sign is marked; if the rate is equal to or greater than baseline or if an interruption occurred, then the minus sign is marked. This process is repeated for each successive minute of the observation period, designated by columns on the BRS Score Sheet.

Calculating the BRS Score

The BRS score for each observation period is the percentage of behaviors scored as relaxed divided by the total number of observations (number of relaxed and unrelaxed behaviors). The number of relaxed behaviors is the total number of plus signs that were circled; the number of unrelaxed behaviors is the number of minus signs circled. If a five-minute observation period is employed, then the total number of observations is 50 (5 minutes x 10 behaviors); if a 10-minute period is employed, then the total number of observations is 100. The BRS may be scored in either a negative (percentage unrelaxed) or positive (percentage relaxed) direction. "Percentage unrelaxed" is the total number of minus signs divided by the total number of observations; "percentage relaxed" is the total number of plus signs divided by the total number of observations. Negative scoring may be used to show a decline in unrelaxed behavior parallel to decreases in muscle tension.[33] Positive scoring shows progress in a fashion more easily understood by the participant and is the most frequently used method to display BRS data. The trainer should choose a scoring method that best serves the requirement of the particular training session.

Baseline Breathing Rate

A baseline rate must be established as the standard against which further breathing rates are measured. It is important to observe a sufficient number of intervals to obtain a representative sample of breathing rates. For research studies, we recommend a minimum of three five-minute observation periods, a total of fifteen measurement intervals. Depending on the clinical setting, a single baseline session of fifteen minutes, in which the participant is told to relax as he or she normally does, may be sufficient.

During baseline observation sessions, breathing is scored as described previously. The mean rate is then calculated by summing all the individual rates for each interval and dividing by the total number of observations. Intervals that were scored as "interruptions" are not included in calculating the mean breathing rate. Any fractional value for the mean breathing rate is rounded up to the next whole number. This value is then entered in the box at the top of the BRS Score Sheet as the Baseline Breathing Rate. The astute reader will have observed that the BRS score for baseline sessions cannot be calculated until after a mean baseline breathing rate has been determined. Once the baseline breathing rate has been established, the BRS score for baseline sessions can then be calculated in the same way as it is for other sessions.

Training BRS Observers

The trainer wishing to use the BRS must be able to do so easily and accurately. Ease of use allows the BRS to be unobtrusively incorporated into the relaxation training routine. Accuracy is essential to make sure that the BRS does the job it is intended to do. In addition, when the BRS is employed in research settings, it is important to demonstrate that it is scored reliably, that is, that two or more observers observe and report the same events. In this regard, Boice[46] reported that investigators employing behavioral observation routinely fail to evaluate the competence of their observers. Simply requiring observers to produce similar reports does not ensure accuracy or reliability. Training observers is itself an issue in behavioral technology.[47]

On its face, the BRS appears straightforward and simple to learn and use. But this simplicity should not mislead the user into assuming that no observer training is necessary. It does, however, make such training relatively easy to accomplish. With undergraduate and graduate students, we have found the following training protocol, based on behavioral technology principles[47,48] to be effective in training observers to accurately and reliably use the BRS.

MASTERY OF DEFINITIONS AND SCORING. First, the observers must master the definitions of each of the ten relaxed behaviors and unrelaxed behaviors, described previously. In addition, the use of the BRS Score Sheet must be mastered. After memorizing the items, observers should pass a written test covering all BRS items. Observers are required to name the 10 relaxed behaviors and then provide the definition of each. Sample tests are provided in Appendix D. A 100 percent criterion of proficiency is recommended before proceeding with training.

Analog Relaxation Observation

Observers are now ready to score the items of the BRS with a live or video-recorded model. If facilities permit, and if many observers need to be trained, then it is useful to construct a recording that provides a standardized sequence of behaviors to be scored.

INDIVIDUAL ITEMS. For successive thirty-second intervals, the observer monitors a single item of the BRS and scores it as relaxed or unrelaxed. A predetermined sequence of items is followed. The model (live or recorded) emits relaxed behavior during a random 50 percent of the intervals and various unrelaxed behaviors during the other 50 percent. In addition to learning discrimination of the behaviors, this procedure trains the observer to keep track of time while observing the model. Practice should continue until 100 percent proficiency is achieved.

MULTIPLE ITEMS. A five-minute observation period is employed in which the observer scores successive one-minute intervals for all ten items on the BRS, using the BRS Score Sheet. The model displays a predetermined sequence of relaxed and unrelaxed behaviors. Video recorded demonstrations are particularly useful at this stage in that a series of five-minute scenes can be employed and the observer's score compared to the predetermined standard. If the scenes are done live, then the model must be skillful in following the predetermined sequence so that questions do not arise as to whether the model or observer was responsible for the disagreement. If live observation is employed, then it is best to have a trained primary observer simultaneously score the intervals and serve as a standard of comparison. Each of the fifty cells in the BRS Score Sheet for a five-minute observation period is compared to the standard, and disagreements are explained. A video recording is useful in this regard because an interval in question can be replayed and differences in opinion resolved.

LIVE RELAXATION OBSERVATION. If video recording has been employed in the previous step, then observation of a live model is now necessary. Comparisons of the observer's BRS scoring to a trained primary observer's scoring are carried out, and inter-observer agreement (IOA) is calculated. IOA is expressed as a percentage in which the number of agreements between two observers divided by fifty (for a five-minute period) and multiplied by one hundred. Training should continue until reliability is consistently 90 percent or better. Disagreements should be discussed and clarified.

Not all technicians or implementers will be graduate students with advanced observational skills. Registered Behavioral Technicians are increasingly being called upon to perform complex observations and interventions. Acquisition of direct observation skills by these individuals can be challenging[49] and more systematic shaping and fading procedures may be needed.

OBSERVATION OF A PARTICIPANT. The observer can now score an actual participant in conjunction with another trained observer. Permission to include another observer should be obtained from the participant, providing the straightforward explanation that the new observer is learning clinical procedures. Agreement between observers should be 90 percent or better. The observer is now ready to serve as an independent or primary observer.

RECALIBRATION. Many authors have recommended that observers periodically undergo a check of their observation skills during the course of a project to guard against "observer drift."[48] Observers occasionally can be cycled through the previous two steps for this purpose.

In conclusion, researchers and practitioners are encouraged to evaluate the effectiveness of this or any observer training program. In addition, research reports should include the results of such evaluations and a description of observer training procedures with sufficient detail for replication.

Validation of the BRS

Validation of an assessment device or procedure requires the demonstration of correspondence between scores on that device and some other accepted criterion of behavior. *Discriminant validity* of a measure is demonstrated when individuals who have met some training criterion score differently on the measure than people who do not meet criterion or who have not been trained at all. In this instance, BRS scores should discriminate people who have undergone relaxation training from those who have not. *Construct validity* is demonstrated when scores on the assessment device are systematically related to other measures of the target behavior. In the present case, BRS scores can be related to other measures of relaxation, such as self-report, physiological measures, or expert opinion. The BRS has been validated in both instances.

DISCRIMINANT VALIDITY OF THE BRS. Schilling and Poppen[38] trained groups of young adults who volunteered for a stress-management program using four procedures: frontalis EMG biofeedback, PMR, BRT, and a music placebo. Everyone received seven training sessions as well as pre- and post-training assessments, and all training was conducted in individual sessions. Biofeedback consisted of auditory feedback from changes in frontalis tension. PMR consisted of audiotaped tense-release exercise instructions of Bernstein and colleagues.[44] BRT consisted of training in the specific postures related to the BRS (see Chapter 4). Music consisted of taped presentations of music commercially marketed as a stress reduction aid, along with attention-focusing instructions. Each of the three relaxation procedures resulted in statistically significant improvements in frontalis EMG and BRS scores, whereas the placebo procedure did not. These effects are seen in Figure 3.1 and 3.2. Direct instruction in the items of the BRS resulted in the greatest change, but statistically significant improvements also occurred for those receiving PMR and biofeedback. By contrast, people administered the placebo condition showed no systematic improvement on the BRS.

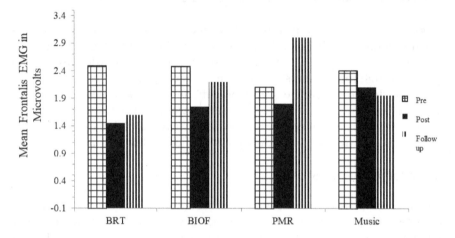

Figure 3.1. Mean EMG in microvolts for each experimental condition at pre-, post-, and follow up assessment.

Based on Schilling, D.J. & Poppen, R. (1983). Behavioral relaxation training and assessment. *Journal of Behavior Therapy and Experimental Psychiatry, 14,* 99–107.

Independent verification of this finding was reported by Norton et al.[35] They compared two groups of college student participants who expressed interest in stress management. One group received two weekly sessions of audiotaped PMR[44] along with a copy of the tape and instructions to practice daily. Those in a control group were instructed to "relax as you best know how." A variety of physiological and self-report measures were obtained before and after the training period. These researchers found a statistically significant improvement on the BRS, from less than 30 percent to approximately 40 percent relaxed, for the relaxation group, whereas no change occurred in the control group. By comparison, Schilling and Poppen[38] found much higher relaxation scores before and after training than did Norton et al.[50] (approximately from 78 percent to 87 percent relaxed for the PMR group).

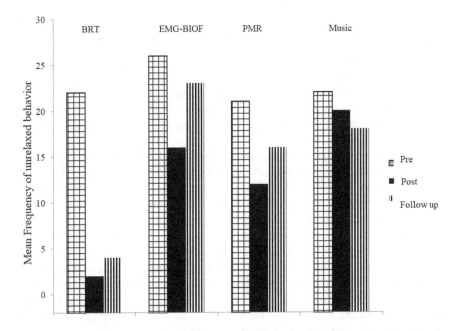

Figure 3.2 Mean Behavioral Relaxation Scale (BRS) (unrelaxed) scores for Behavioral Relaxation Training (BRT), frontalis electromyography biofeedback (BIOF), progressive relaxation (PMR), and music placebo (MUSIC).

Based on Schilling, D.J. & Poppen, R. (1983). Behavioral relaxation training and assessment. *Journal of Behavior Therapy and Experimental Psychiatry, 14*, 99–107.

Blanchard and colleagues,[50] as part of a hypertension treatment program, reported that participants receiving PMR training sessions achieved an average of 84 percent relaxed behaviors on the BRS for their last four training sessions. Unfortunately, neither pre-treatment BRS measures nor BRS measures for participants in a thermal biofeedback group were collected. In a later report, this research group found that BRS scores steadily improved from about 70 percent to better than 80 percent over eight sessions of training in PMR.[51] These figures are comparable with those of Schilling and Poppen.[38]

Luiselli[20] described a Relaxation Checklist similar in many respects to the BRS. He reported that significant increases in relaxed behavior occurred on this checklist for college students who received a single PMR session, whereas those receiving a control procedure showed no change.

In summary, discriminant validity of the BRS was demonstrated by three separate research groups in which training in PMR resulted in improved BRS scores. More training appeared to produce more improvements, and no training or placebo procedure resulted in no systematic change. One study also found that frontalis EMG biofeedback resulted in increased relaxed behavior on the BRS. According to the four-modality response system model presented in Chapter 2, the BRS measures primarily motor behavior; PMR and EMG biofeedback are primarily motor procedures, thus, a strong association would be expected. If relaxation comprises a response class across modalities, then one would expect that training procedures emphasizing verbal, visceral, or observational modalities also would result in improved BRS scores. Demonstration of this relationship awaits further research.

CONSTRUCT VALIDITY OF THE BRS. The BRS also has been validated by concurrent measures of relaxation. Schilling and Poppen[38] found significant correlations between frontalis EMG levels and the BRS, particularly in the BRT and biofeedback groups. The BRS was not related to visceral measures of skin temperature or skin conductance.

Norton et al.[35] also found a significant correlation between the BRS and heart rate and respiration rate, even when the breathing item was removed from the BRS so as not to spuriously inflate the relationship. Their relaxation training and control groups did not differ on physiological measures; both improved over time. Wittrock et al.[51] found a significant correlation between BRS scores and decreased systolic blood pressure in hypertensive participants during the last two sessions of PMR training.

In a direct validation study, Poppen and Maurer[52] measured EMG levels in the muscles anatomically related to the postures described in the BRS. Six male volunteers, ages 23 to 27 years, served as participants. EMG measurements were collected as the participants engaged in the relaxed or unrelaxed postures for five-minute periods. Participants were not instructed to "tense" or "relax," but rather were instructed and guided into the postures as topographically described in the BRS. In all instances, EMG levels for relaxed postures were significantly lower than those for unrelaxed postures. Tension in the forearm extensors in this muscle group was equally elevated while participants extended or flexed their fingers. Similarly, tension in the forearm flexors was elevated in both extended and flexed unrelaxed postures. EMG levels for unilateral sternocleidomastoid while the head was rotated in a contralateral direction, to the side opposite the electrode placement, were greater than those during ipsilateral rotation. Tension levels in the gracillis muscle group of the upper right thigh was higher when the feet were parallel, with the toes pointed up, than when the toes were pointed out about 90 degrees. The opposite was true for the vastus muscle group. Tension levels in the trapezius were elevated when the shoulders were slightly raised. Tension in the suprahyoid muscles were elevated when the shoulders were slightly raised, and also increased while participants engaged in one -minute intervals of: (a) talking; (b) coughing; (c) swallowing; (d) clearing their throats; and, (e) humming. Tension in the masseter muscle of the jaw was elevated while participants (a) placed their lips and teeth together, and it increased even more while participants (b) engaged in smiling. Tension in the canthus area of the eye was elevated when the eyes were open. Tension increased even more when the eyelids were closed but (a) the eyelids were fluttering; (b) the eyelids were squeezed; and, (c) the eyes were moving under the eyelids.

The study by Poppen and Maurer[52] effectively dissected the BRS, showing that each item is intimately related to tension levels in the relevant muscle groups. Thus, when a person assumes a related posture, tension in the associated muscle groups decreases markedly. As people undergo relaxation training (by whatever procedure) and learn to minimize tension throughout their bodies, this is reflected by the relaxed behaviors defined by the BRS.

The relationship between verbal self-reports and BRS is complicated by the fact that verbal reports of calmness often accompany a credible training procedure irrespective of other measures of relaxation. Schilling and Poppen[38] found that participants in all groups—placebo as well as relaxation—reported increased subjective feelings of relaxation; these reports were not related to BRS scores or EMG levels. Likewise, Norton et al.[35] found that both relaxation training and control groups improved to a similar extent on a number of verbal inventories, including scales of state anxiety, state anger, stress, and arousal, as well as the visual analog scale for relaxation. However, they also found that improvements on all these measures except "stress" were correlated with improvements on the BRS. Wittrock et al.[51] did not calculate correlations between self-ratings of relaxation and the BRS, but their data indicated that both scores increased in a similar fashion over training sessions and that, like the BRS, self-ratings were correlated with blood pressure only in the last two sessions.

Additional research has been conducted using the BRS as a process or outcome measure in applied and experimental research, further validating its utility. Scheufele[53] employed a modified Upright BRS to assess relaxed behavior in three experimental conditions: (a) PMR; (b) music; and, (c) silence. Upright BRS scores were significantly higher for the PMR group. These results replicate and extend those of Norton[35] to the extent that the UBRS was shown to be a valid measure of relaxation. Suhr, Anderson and Tranel[54] employed the BRS to assess the effects of PMR used to reduce the challenging behavior of older adults with mild to moderate Alzheimer's disease. Unfortunately, no measures of relaxed behavior were reported in relation to the decline in challenging behavior reported. Chan, Chien, and To[55] used the BRS as part of a randomized controlled trial evaluating the effect of multisensory intervention for individuals with intellectual disabilities. Significant differences in BRS scores were obtained at the end of treatment.

To summarize, construct validity of the BRS has been shown by appropriate changes in concurrent measures of relaxation, particularly EMG levels. Tension in the relevant musculature is closely related to relaxed and unrelaxed postures as defined by the BRS. Correlations between the BRS and visceral measures of heart rate, respiration rate, and blood pressure have been reported, but correlation with skin temperature and skin conductance has not been found. Some relationship between BRS and self-report has been found, but self-report of relaxation often improves over time regardless of training procedure or other measures.

CONCLUSION

Although relaxation training methods have been employed for decades, the status of relaxation as a scientific construct is very recent. A major reason has been the lack of an objective measurement system for what is widely assumed to be a subjective state. Some professionals have learned to live with this state of affairs and have focused instead on measuring the relation between treatment procedure and symptom change, whereas others have made do with approximate measures of relaxation. This chapter proposes that measuring relaxation enhances the assessment of treatment outcome. The BRS is presented as an objective method for measuring the motor component of relaxation, along with evidence for its reliability and validity. This method is placed in the context of a multimodal conceptualization of relaxation. We regard the BRS as a crucial, but by no means complete, metric. It is available to stimulate further research on the assessment of relaxation and to aid in the development of more effective training procedures.

REFERENCES

[1]Gutkin, A. J., Holborn, S. W., Walker, J. R., & Anderson, B. A. (1992). Treatment integrity of relaxation training for tension headaches. *Journal of Behavior Therapy and Experimental Psychiatry, 23*, 191–198. https://doi.org/10.1016/0005-7916(92)90036-I

[2]Yeaton, W. H., & Sechrest, L. (1981). Critical dimensions in the choice and maintenance of successful treatments: Strength, integrity, and effectiveness. *Journal of Consulting and Clinical Psychology, 49*, 156–167. https://doi.org/10.1037/0022-006X.49.2.156

[3]Perepletchikova, F., & Kazdin, A. E. (2005). Treatment integrity and therapeutic change: Issues and research recommendations. *Clinical Psychology: Science and Practice, 12*, 365–383. https://doi.org/10.1093/clipsy.bpi045

[4]Wheeler, J. J., Baggett, B. A., Fox, J., & Blevins, L. (2006). Treatment integrity. A review of intervention studies conducted with children with autism. *Focus Autism*

Other Developmental Disabilities, 21, 45–54. https://doi.org/10.1177/10883576060210010601

[5]Wilder, D. A., Atwell, J., & Wine, B. (2006). The effects of varying levels of treatment integrity on child compliance during treatment with a three-step prompting procedure. *Journal of Applied Behavior Analysis, 39*, 369–373. https://doi.org/10.1901/jaba.2006.144-05

[6]Hillenberg, J. B., & Collins, F. L., Jr. (1982). A procedural analysis and review of relaxation training research. *Behavior Research and Therapy, 20*, 251–260. https://doi.org/10. 1016/0005-7967(82)90143-7

[7]Skinner, B. F. (1953). *Science and human behavior*. New York: McMillan.

[8]Ferster, C. B. (1965). Classification of behavior pathology. In L. Krasner, & L. Ullman (Eds.), *Research in behavior modification*. NY: Holt, Rhinehart and Winston.

[9]Kanfer, F. H., & Saslow, G. (1965). Behavioral analysis. An alternative to diagnostic classification. *Archives of General Psychiatry, 12*, 329–538. https://doi.org/10.1001/archpsyc. 1965.01720360001001

[10]Cone, J. D. (1979). Issues in functional analysis in behavioral assessment. *Behavior Research and Therapy, 35*, 259–275. https://doi.org/10.1016/S0005-7967(96)00101-5

[11]Iwata, B. A., Dorsey, M. F., Slifer, K. J., Bauman, K. E., & Richman, G. S. (1994). Toward a functional analysis of self-injury. *Journal of Applied Behavior Analysis, 27*(2), 197–209. https://doi.org/10.1901/jaba.1994.27-197

[12]Kiesel, K. B., Lutzker, J. R., & Cambell, R. V. (1989). Behavioral relaxation Training to reduce hyperventilation and seizures in a profoundly retarded epileptic child. *Journal of the Multihandicapped Person, 2*, 179–190. https://doi.org/10.1007/BF01100089

[13]Harris, R. (2008). *Clarifying your values (Adapted from Tobias Lundgren's Bull's eye Worksheet)*. Retrieved February 24, 2019 from https://thehappinesstrap.com/upimages/Long_Bull%27s_Eye_Worksheet.pdf.

[14]Skinner, B. F. (1969*). Contingencies of reinforcement: A theoretical analysis*. NY: Appleton-Century-Crofts.

[15]Zettle, R., & Hayes, S. C. (1984). Rule-governed behavior: A potential theoretical framework for cognitive behavior therapy. In P. C. Kendall (Ed.), *Advances in cognitive-behavioral research and therapy*, Volume 1 (pp. 73–118). NY: Academic Press.

[16]Wolpe, J. (1958). *Psychotherapy by reciprocal inhibition*. Stanford, CA: Stanford University Press.

[17]Schilling, D. J., & Poppen, R. (1983). Behavioral relaxation training and assessment. *Journal of Behavior Therapy and Experimental Psychiatry, 14*, 99–107. https://doi.org/10. 1016/0005-7916(83)90027-7

[18]Lehrer, P. M., Carr, R., Sargunaraj, D., & Woolfolk, R. L. (1994). Stress management techniques: Are they all equivalent or do they have specific effects? *Biofeedback and Self-Regulation, 19*, 353–401. https://doi.org/10.1007/BF01776735

[19]Luiselli, J. K. (1980). Relaxation training with the developmentally disabled: A reappraisal. *Behavior Research with Severe Developmental Disabilities, 1*, 191–213. https://doi.org/10.1016/S0005-7894(79)80068-4

[20]Luiselli, J. K., Marholin, D., Steinman, D. L., & Steinman, W. M. (1979). Assessing the effects of relaxation training. *Behavior Therapy, 10*, 663–668. https://doi.org/10.1016/S0005-7894(79)80068-4

[21]Crist, D. A., & Rickard, H. C. (1993). A "fair" comparison of progressive and imaginal relaxation. *Perceptual and Motor Skills, 76,* 691–700. https://doi.org/10.2466/pms.1993.76.2.691

[22]Crist, D. A., Rickard, H. C., Prentice-Dunn, S., & Barker, H. R. (1989). The Relaxation Inventory: Self-report scales of relaxation training effects. *Journal of Personality Assessment, 53,* 716–726. https://doi.org/10.1207/s15327752jpa5304_872

[23]Hites, L. S., & Lundervold, D. A. (2013). Relation between direct observation of relaxed behavior and self-reported mindfulness and relaxation. *International Journal of Behavioral Consultation and Therapy, 7,* 6–7. https://doi.org/10.1037/h0100958

[24]Smith, J. C., Amutio, A., Anderson, J. P., & Aria, L. A. (1996). Relaxation: Mapping an uncharted world. *Biofeedback and Self-Regulation, 21,* 63–90. https://doi.org/10.1007/BF02214150

[25]Smith, J. C. (1999). *ABC relaxation theory. An evidence-based approach.* NY: Springer.

[26]Smith, J. C. (2001). *Advances in ABC relaxation: Applications and inventories.* NY: Springer.

[27]Smith, J. C. (2005). *Relaxation, Meditation, and Mindfulness.* NY: Springer.

[28]Hobbs, C. (2009). *Effect of Behavioral Relaxation Training on self-reported relaxation states and mindfulness.* Unpublished master's thesis. University of Central Missouri.

[29]Roemer, L. (2003). Mindfulness: A promising intervention strategy in need of further study. *Clinical Psychology: Science and Practice, 10,* 172–178. https://doi.org/10.1093/clipsy.bpg020

[30]Baer, R. A., Smith, G. T., Hopkins, J., Krietemeyer, J., & Toney, L. (2006). Using self-report assessment methods to explore facets of mindfulness. *Assessment, 13,* 27–45. https://doi.org/10.1177/1073191105283504

[31]Lettow, L., Hites, L. S., & Lundervold, D. A. (2012). *States of arousal and relaxation: Empirical analysis of dimensions of relaxation.* Association for Psychological Science, Chicago, IL.

[32]Lundervold, D. A., Kopp, R., Garcia, A., Fontanette, T., & Ament, P. A. (2014). *States of arousal and relaxation (STAR) questionnaire measures mindfulness.* Association for Psychological Science, San Francisco, CA.

[33]Lau, M., A., Bishop, S. R., Segal, Z. V., Buis, T., Anderson, N. D., Carlson, L., Shapiro, S., & Carmody, J. (2006). The Toronto Mindfulness Scale: Development and validation. *Journal of Clinical Psychology, 62,* 1445–1467. https://doi.org/10.1002/jclp.20326

[34]Mathews, A. M. (1971). Psychophysiological approaches to the investigation of desensitization and related procedures. *Psychological Bulletin, 76,* 73–91. https://doi.org/10.1037/h0031479

[35]Norton, M., Holm, J. E., & McSherry, W. C., II. (1997). Behavioral assessment of relaxation: The validity of a behavioral rating scale. *Journal of Behavior Therapy and Experimental Psychiatry, 28,* 129–137. https://doi.org/10.1016/S0005-7916(97)00004-9

[36]Qualls, P. J., & Sheehan, P. W. (1981). Electromyographic biofeedback as a relaxation training technique: A critical appraisal and reassessment. *Psychological Bulletin, 90,* 21–42. https://doi.org/10.1037/0033-2909.90.1.21

[37]Reinking, R. H., & Hutchings, D. (1981). Follow-up to: "Tension headaches: what form of therapy is most effective?" *Biofeedback and Self-Regulation, 6,* 57–62. https://doi.org/10.1007/BF00998793

[38]Schilling, D. J., & Poppen, R. (1983). Behavioral relaxation training and assessment. *Journal of Behavior Therapy and Experimental Psychiatry, 14*, 99–107. https://doi.org/ 10.1016/ 0005-7916(83)90027-7

[39]Taylor, D. N., & Lee, C. T. (1991). Lack of correlation between frontalis electromyography and self-ratings of either frontalis tension or state anxiety. *Perceptual and Motor Skills, 72*, 1131–1134. https://doi.org/10.2466/pms.1991.72.3c.

[40]Blanchard, E. B., & Andrasik, F. (1985). *Management of chronic headaches*. New York: Pergamon.

[41]Fordyce, W. (1976). *Behavioral methods for chronic pain and illness*. St. Louis, MO: Mosby.

[42]Jacobson, E. (1938). *Progressive relaxation*. Chicago: University of Chicago Press. (Originally published 1929).

[43]Wolpe, J., & Lazarus, A. A. (1966). *Behavior therapy techniques: A guide to the treatment of neuroses*. Oxford, UK: Pergamon.

[44]Bernstein, D. A., Borkovec, T. D., & Hazlett- Stevens, H. (2000). *New directions in progressive relaxation training: A guidebook for helping professionals*. Westport CT: Praeger Publishers.

[45]Lundervold, D. A., & Dunlap, A. L. (2006). Alternate forms reliability of the Behavioral Relaxation Scale: Preliminary results. *International Journal of Behavioral Consultation and Therapy, 2*, 240–245. https://doi.org/10.1037/h0100779

[46]Boice, R. (1983). Observational skills. *Psychological Bulletin, 93*, 3–29. https://doi.org/10.1037/0033-2909.93.1.3

[47]Johnston, J. M., & Pennypacker, H. S. (2009). *Strategies and tactics of human behavioral research*. (3rd ed.) Hillsdale, NJ: Lawrence Erlbaum.

[48]Foster, S. L., & Cone, J. D. (1986). Design and use of direct observation methods. In A. R. Ciminero, K. S. Calhoun, & H. E. Adams (Eds.), *Handbook of behavioral assessment, 2nd ed*. (pp. 253–324). New York: John Wiley.

[49]Walkup, A. (2017). *Personal communication with the first author*.

[50]Blanchard, E. B., McCoy, G. C., Musso, A., Gerardi, M. A., Pallmever, T. P., Gerardi, R. J., Cotch, P. A., Siracusa, K., & Andrasik, F. (1986). A controlled comparison of thermal biofeedback and relaxation training in the treatment of essential hypertension: I. Short-term and long-term outcome. *Behavior Therapy, 17*, 563–579. https://doi.org/10.1016/S0005-7894(86)80095-8

[51]Wittrock, D. A., Blanchard, E. B., & McCoy, G. C. (1988). Three studies on the relation of process to outcome in the treatment of essential hypertension. *Behavior Research and Therapy, 26*, 53–66. https://doi.org/10.1016/0005-7967(88)90033-2

[52]Poppen, R., & Maurer, J. (1982). Electromyographic analysis of relaxed postures. *Biofeedback and Self-Regulation, 7*, 491–498. https://doi.org/10.1007/BF00998889

[53]Scheufele, P. M. (2000). Effects of progressive relaxation and classical music on measurements of attention, relaxation and stress responses. *Journal of Behavioral Medicine, 23*, 207–228. https://doi.org/10.1023/A:1005542121935

[54]Suhr, J., Anderson, S., & Tranel, D. (1999). Progressive muscle relaxation in the management of behavioral disturbance in Alzheimer's Disease. *Neuropsychological Rehabilitation, 9*, 31–44. https://doi.org/10.1080/713755590

[55]Chan, S. W. C., Chien, W. T., & To, M. Y. F. (2007). An evaluation of the clinical effectiveness of a multisensory therapy on individuals with learning disability. *Hong Kong Medical Journal, 13*, (Suppl 1): S28–31.

Supplement
Behavior Analyst Certification Board 5th Edition Task List

B. Concepts and Principles
B-1 Define and provide examples of behavior, response, and response class.
B-8 Define and provide examples of unconditioned, conditioned, and generalized reinforcers and punishers.

C. Measurement, Data Display, and Interpretation
C-1 Establish operational definitions of behavior.
C-2 Distinguish among direct, indirect, and product measures of behavior.
C-3 Measure occurrence (e.g., frequency, rate, percentage).
C-5 Measure form and strength of behavior (e.g., topography, magnitude).
C-7 Design and implement sampling procedures (i.e., interval recording, time sampling).
C-8 Evaluate the validity and reliability of measurement procedures.
C-9 Select a measurement system to obtain representative data given the dimensions of behavior and the logistics of observing and recording.
C-10 Graph data to communicate relevant quantitative relations (e.g., equal-interval graphs, bar graphs, cumulative records).

G. Behavior-Change Procedures
G-1 Use positive and negative reinforcement procedures to strengthen behavior.

I. Personnel Supervision and Management
I-4 Train personnel to competently perform assessment and intervention procedures.

Chapter 4
Behavioral Relaxation Training Procedures

This chapter presents the standard Behavioral Relaxation Training (BRT) procedure for use with adults and older children who have "normal" learning capabilities. It is indicated for persons having various stress, pain, or anxiety disorders for which relaxation, in a generic sense, is often employed. The present chapter describes some preconditions for BRT, gives a step-by-step explanation of the training method, describes some variations and extensions of BRT, and discusses problems that may arise in the course of training. BRT procedures for special populations are presented in subsequent chapters.

As discussed in Chapter 2, BRT has many features in common with other relaxation training methods that make it useful as an intervention in the wide range of problems for which relaxation is prescribed. In addition, BRT has characteristics that may make it preferable to other training methods. First is the relative ease and rapidity of acquiring relaxed behaviors. Although achieving proficiency and employing relaxation in everyday situations takes additional time and practice, participants usually are able to begin the process with a high level of success that sets the stage for continuing progress. Also, variations of BRT, termed *upright relaxation*, *mini-relaxation*, and *focused breathing*, make it highly portable and easily implemented in everyday situations.

Compared to other training methods, BRT has additional advantages. Unlike PMR, it does not require muscle contraction, which may be contraindicated for problems related to muscle tension, such as tension headache and myofacial pain. And unlike meditation and imagery procedures, it is easy for both trainer and participant to monitor acquisition of target behavior. Chapter 5 provides more extensive comparisons of BRT and other relaxation training methods, and describes in detail its clinical applications.

PREREQUISITES FOR TRAINING

When introducing a participant to BRT, there are several preliminary considerations. These include assessing problematic behaviors, providing a rationale for learning relaxation skills as an antidote to these problems, clarifying expectations about participant practice, and arranging a setting for training.

Assessment of Problem Behaviors

Several indirect behavioral assessment procedures are generally useful. (More specific assessment methods will be described in subsequent chapters for particular disorders.) These include a clinical interview to obtain the participant's history, reviewing medical records, use of values clarification exercise and brief motivational interviewing need to be addressed as discussed in Chapter 3.[1]

The Rationale for BRT

The rationale flows directly from assessment, providing reasons why the participant should follow the trainer's instructions. These "rules for relaxation" state the relationships among antecedents, behaviors, and consequences of relaxation. The specifics of this general formula are as varied as the individuals who can benefit from relaxation training, and no universal prescription is provided here. In general, the following steps are useful in developing and presenting a rationale: (a) review the problematic behavior; (b) clarification of the participant's values for living; (c) use of brief motivational interviewing to set the occasion for overt talk of behavior change and identification of reinforcers of behavior change; (d) clarification of the treatment goal; (e) present relaxation as an effective alternative response; and, (f) describe the training procedure.[2-4]

In short, relaxation is proposed as an effective alternative to problem behavior. Often, a structural explanation is useful in which the physiological aspects of relaxation are described as overriding the problematic condition. Such explanations are variations of Wolpe's[5] incompatibility or "reciprocal inhibition hypothesis" in which relaxation is held to be physically incompatible with the problem state, be it "anxiety," "stress," "arousal," or "poor concentration." A functional explanation also can be employed in which relaxed behavior is presented as effective in gaining desired outcomes. For example, by relaxing the eyes, jaw, and shoulders, a headache participant may reduce tension and prevent pain.[6] Or, by sitting quietly and observing slow, regular breathing, a hyperactive child may do assignments more efficiently and gain the teacher's approval.

Whatever the mechanism, the rationale emphasizes the reinforcing consequences (positive and negative reinforcement) of engaging in relaxed behavior, although care should be taken not to imply a guaranteed benefit. No procedure has been found to be 100 percent effective, and the trainer should make an "educated guess" based on the literature on BRT and related techniques. However, more than three decades of research across the lifespan and myriad target behaviors, BRT has been shown to be an evidence-based treatment with a high likelihood of benefit.

Commitment to Practice

Finally, the training procedure, along with expected time and practice commitments, is described. BRT is presented as a skill in which proficiency comes with practice. Although the relaxed postures themselves usually are learned very quickly, beneficial outcomes result from regular practice and from implementation throughout the day. The therapist and participant need to discuss what facilities are available for practice in the home and other environments, and what times are most amenable. They can problem-solve in making practice arrangements and dealing with changes as training and implementation progress.

The Setting

The physical and social environments for training should be conducive to relaxation. As discussed in Chapter 2, for the participant to observe the low intensity events of interest, distracting and interrupting stimuli must be minimized. Lighting may be dimmed to provide a relaxing atmosphere, but it should be sufficient to allow observation of the participant's behavior. External noise, such as loud talk in the waiting room, should be prevented. And the usual strictures regarding cell phones apply.

Full bodily support should be provided so that the participant need not exert effort to maintain his or her posture. A padded reclining chair with footrest is routinely employed, but care should be taken that the participant fits the chair comfortably. Small pillows can be used to fill gaps that may occur beneath the participant's elbows or lower back. If training or practice is done on a flat surface such as a floor or bed, then pillows should be placed beneath the participant's knees, forearms, and head, flexing the legs, arms, and spine slightly. This flattens the spine and prevents discomfort from lordosis. We have found a beanbag chair to be useful for small children, and this also may be acceptable for adults. The seating position for the trainer, to allow adequate observation of the participant's behavior, was described in Chapter 3.

ACQUISITION TRAINING PROCEDURES

After presenting the rationale, answering questions, and gaining the cooperation of the participant, training is ready to commence.

Organization of Training Sessions

A BRT session is typically 45 to 50 minutes, though what is accomplished is based on the context and rate of acquisition of the participant. Table 4.1 shows the recommended time intervals for each phase.

An initial adaptation period, in which the participant is asked to sit quietly with his or her eyes closed, allows the participant to "shift gears" from the previous activities of the day to the task of learning relaxed behaviors. Adaptation is particularly important if physiologic measures are to be recorded.

Pre-training baseline observations, described in Chapter 3, allow assessment of the participant's progress over successive sessions. During baseline assessment, the participant is asked to relax while the trainer scores the behavior using the Behavioral Relaxation Scale (BRS) Recording Form and collects a self-report at the conclusion of the observation period.

During acquisition training, the relaxed behaviors are trained by means of description, modeling, guidance, and feedback. Usually, for participants without serious disabilities or impaired functioning, initial acquisition can be accomplished within two sessions. The time required varies, of course, depending on the individual participant.

In proficiency training, the participant practices the relaxed postures with feedback from the trainer. The feedback is primarily verbal, although modeling and guidance are used if necessary. The duration of a proficiency training session may be adjusted to meet the needs of the participant. Some

Table 4.1
General Outline of Behavioral Relaxation Training
Session Time Recommendations

Phase	Time required (minutes)
Adaptation	5–10
Pre-training observation	5
Aquisition training (first session only)	15–20
Proficiency training	15–30
Post-training observation	5

people, especially early in training, find it difficult to sit still for extended periods. This and other problems encountered in training are discussed in later sections.

The post-training observation period provides a BRS score that, in comparison to the baseline score, indicates progress in that session. It also provides a measure of relaxation over successive training sessions.

Relaxed Behavior Training Sequence

The ten relaxed behaviors listed in the BRS may be taught in any order, but we have developed a logical sequence that seems to work best for both trainer and participant. *Body* is taught first because placement of the torso in the recliner is the basic foundation for all the rest. Then a head-to-toe pattern is followed that aligns the major muscle groups: *Head, Shoulders, Hands, Feet*. Next, the smaller muscle groups are trained: *Throat, Quiet, Breathing, Mouth,* and *Eyes*. Eyes are last so that the participant can visually observe modeling by the trainer, and closed eyes provide a natural segue into the post-training assessment period.

Some people can learn all ten behaviors in a single session. If two or more acquisition sessions are required, the first five items comprise a natural grouping, with the next five taught on subsequent sessions.

Initial Training Steps

Initial acquisition involves four steps for each of the ten behaviors. These steps are as follows.

1. **Labeling**. Each behavior is given a one-word label by which it can be conveniently identified (i.e. body, head, shoulders, hands, feet, throat, quiet, breathing, mouth, eyes).
2. **Description and modeling**. Each relaxed behavior is described and demonstrated by the trainer. Commonly occurring unrelaxed behaviors also are demonstrated and the contrast with relaxed behavior is pointed out.
3. **Imitation**. The participant is asked to demonstrate the relaxed posture.
4. **Feedback**. The participant is praised for correct imitation. If they do not display the proper posture, then the trainer first provides corrective verbal instructions. If after two or three such prompts the participant still is unsuccessful, then manual guidance is gently employed to move the participant into the correct position. When success is achieved, positive feedback is given.

Cumulative Performance

As each behavior is successfully acquired, the participant is asked to maintain the posture or activity for 30 to 60 seconds and to observe the feelings that occur. They also are asked to maintain the trained behaviors as each new one is added. In this way, all ten behaviors are built up gradually. If the participant should slip into an unrelaxed instance of a previously trained behavior, then this should be gently pointed out and corrected. If the participant should become "stuck," unable to imitate or maintain a particular behavior after several prompts and manual guidance, then the trainer should move on to the next item. The trainer should reassure the participant that one does not expect perfection right away and that success comes with practice. Problems that may arise in training are discussed in a later section.

A Script for BRT Acquisition

The following is a suggested script for the initial acquisition session. The trainer should practice the script to fluency, although rote memorization is not necessary. Language should be adapted to be appropriate for age, education, or other special characteristics of the participant.

Note that photographs of relaxed and unrelaxed postures are provided in the description of the Behavioral Relaxation Scale in Chapter 3. Those photos are referred to below.

1. *Body.*

   LABELING. There are ten relaxed postures or activities and we use a one-word label for each. The first relaxed posture is called "body."

   DESCRIPTION AND MODELING. Your body is relaxed when your chest and hips are aligned in the chair, with no movement. [Demonstrate as shown in Photo 3.6A.] Your body is unrelaxed if your torso is crooked, if any part of your back or hips is lifted from the chair, or if there is movement in your torso. [Demonstrate as shown in Photo 3.6B].

   IMITATION. Please relax your body.

   FEEDBACK. [Positive:] Good. Now take a few moments to notice the sensations as you relax your body. Notice how your spine is straight when your hips and chest are lined up. [Corrective:] You seem to be a little twisted to your left. Rotate your chest slightly to the right while keeping your hips still. [Guidance: Manual guidance of a person's torso may be difficult, and social conventions regarding touching a participant's chest or hips should be considered.]

2. *Head.*

LABELING. The next posture is termed "head."

DESCRIPTION AND MODELING. Your head is relaxed when it is resting on the cushion, facing straight in midline. [Demonstrate as shown in Photo 3.1A.] Your head is unrelaxed if it is tilted or turned to either side or tilted up or down. [Demonstrate as shown in Photos 3.1B, C.]

IMITATION. Please relax your head.

FEEDBACK. [Positive:] Good. Now just take a few moments to feel the sensations in your neck as you relax your head. Notice how your head is lined up straight with your body. [Corrective:] That's close, but your head is tilted a little to the right. Can you straighten it? [Guidance:] Your head still is tilted slightly. It is okay if I adjust it so it is straight? [Be sure to ask the participant if it is all right to touch them before providing manual guidance. After correction or guidance, be sure to give positive feedback.]

3. *Shoulders.*

LABELING. The next relaxed posture is termed "shoulders."

DESCRIPTION AND MODELING. Your shoulders are relaxed when they are resting against the chair and are sloped or rounded with the tops in a straight line. [Demonstrate as shown in Photo 3.5A.] They are unrelaxed if they are raised or twisted or if one shoulder is higher than the other. [Demonstrate as shown in Photos 3.5B, C.]

IMITATION. All right, can you demonstrate relaxed shoulders?

FEEDBACK. [Positive:] That's right. Now just relax and observe the feelings in your shoulders. [Corrective:] Your left shoulder appears a little higher than your right one. Lower your left shoulder a bit. [Guidance:] Your shoulders still appear a little crooked. Let me place them in a relaxed position. [Be sure to ask the participant before touching him or her. Arrange the person's shoulders by gentle pressure to raise or lower them. Give positive feedback after correction or guidance.]

4. *Hands.*

LABELING. The next area to relax is called "hands."

DESCRIPTION AND MODELING. Your hands are relaxed when you rest them on the arms of the chair, or in your lap, with the fingers slightly curled into a claw-like position like this. [Demonstrate as shown in Photos 3.7A.] Your hands are not relaxed if the fingers are flat or curled into a ball. [Demonstrate as shown in Photos 3.7C, D.]

IMITATION.   Please demonstrate relaxed hands.

FEEDBACK.   [Positive:] That's good. Now just continue to relax for a few moments and notice how your hands and arms feel in this position. [Corrective:] Not quite. Curl your fingers a little more so that a pencil could pass under your pinky. [Guidance:] That's still not quite it. Here, let me show you. [Again, be sure to inform the participant before touching him or her. Mold the participant's hand into the desired posture. After correction or guidance, be sure to give positive feedback.]

5. *Feet.*

LABELING.   The next posture is called "feet."

DESCRIPTION AND MODELING.   Your feet are relaxed when both heels are resting on the footrest with the toes pointed away from each other in a V position. [Demonstrate as shown in Photo 3.8A.] Your feet are not relaxed if your toes are pointing straight up or turned outward too much, or if your ankles are crossed. [Demonstrate as shown in Photos 3.8B, C, D.]

IMITATION.   Please show me relaxed feet.

FEEDBACK.   [Positive:] That's right. Just continue to relax your feet and notice the feelings in your feet and legs as you do so. [Corrective:] Your toes are pointing straight up too much. Just let your legs and feet flop apart. [Guidance:] Allow me to position your feet properly. [Ask the participant before touching him or her. Place the feet in a "V" of about 90 degrees with the heels a couple inches apart. After correction or guidance, be sure to give positive feedback.]

6. *Throat.*

LABELING.   The next relaxed area is termed "throat."

DESCRIPTION AND MODELING.   Your throat is relaxed when it is quiet and smooth. [Demonstrate as shown in Photo 3.4] It is unrelaxed if there is any movement, muscle twitches, or swallowing. [Demonstrate.]

IMITATION.   Please demonstrate a relaxed throat.

FEEDBACK.   [Positive:] That's good. Notice the feelings in your neck and throat as you relax for the next few moments. [Corrective:] That's okay if you have to swallow occasionally, but then just go back to relaxing your throat. [Guidance: Manual guidance is not applicable to throat.]

7. *Quiet.*

LABELING.   The next activity is called "quiet."

DESCRIPTION AND MODELING. You are quiet when you are not making any noise such as talking, loud sighs, or snores. [Demonstrate sounds.]

IMITATION. All right, please demonstrate quiet for the next few moments.

FEEDBACK. [Positive:] Good. Notice the relaxed feelings in your throat and chest as you quietly relax. [Corrective:] Please don't vocalize as you breathe out. [Guidance: Manual guidance is not applicable to quiet.]

8. *Breathing.*

LABELING. The next relaxed activity is called "breathing."

DESCRIPTION AND MODELING. Your breathing is relaxed when it is slow and regular. [Demonstrate.] It is not relaxed if it is rapid or if there are interruptions such as coughing, yawning, sneezing, sniffing, vocalizations, or the like. [Note: The participant is not told the specific number of breaths that serves as his or her criterion for relaxed breathing. In addition to the rate criterion, the trainer may wish to employ *focused breathing* as described in a later section.]

IMITATION. Please demonstrate relaxed breathing.

FEEDBACK. [Observe the breathing rate for at least one 30-second period and compare it to the baseline rate. If the rate is less than baseline, then provide positive feedback; if it is equal to or greater than the baseline rate, then use correction or guidance.] [Positive:] That's good. Just continue to breathe slowly and regularly. [Corrective:] Please slow your breathing. [Guidance:] Please inhale slowly and deeply when I say "in" and exhale slowly when I say "out." [Pace the participant's breathing so that it is slightly less than baseline rate. Provide positive feedback after correction or guidance.] Additional instruction on *focused breathing* may be helpful for some participants. This is covered in a later section of this chapter.

9. *Mouth.*

LABELING. The next relaxed posture is called "mouth."

DESCRIPTION AND MODELING. Your mouth is relaxed when your teeth are parted and your lips are open in the center like this. [Demonstrate as shown in Photo 3.3A.] Your mouth is unrelaxed if your upper and lower teeth are touching, if your lips are closed, or if you smile or lick your lips. [Demonstrate as shown in Photo 3.3B, C.]

IMITATION. Okay, please show me how to relax your mouth.

FEEDBACK. [Positive:] That's right. Now notice the feelings in your jaw and face as you relax your mouth. [Corrective:] Drop your jaw and let your lips open a little wider. [Guidance: Manual guidance usually is not applicable to mouth.]

10. *Eyes.*

   LABELING.   The final relaxed area is called "eyes."

   DESCRIPTION AND MODELING.   Your eyes are relaxed when the eyelids are closed and smooth. [Demonstrate as shown in Photo 3.2A.] Your eyes are not relaxed when they are open, or if they are tightly shut, or if there is eye movement beneath the eyelids. [Demonstrate as shown in Photo 3.2B, C.]

   IMITATION.   Please relax your eyes.

   FEEDBACK.   [Positive:] That's right. Notice the relaxed feelings in your eyes and forehead as you relax for a few moments. [Corrective:] Your eyelids are closed a little too tightly. Allow them to become smooth. [Guidance: Manual guidance is not applicable to eyes.]

A Script for Reviewing Relaxed Behaviors

After completing all ten items, the trainer should review them, as follows, to aid the participant's recall. Be sure to pause for five to ten seconds between each item and to provide positive or corrective feedback as indicated. The following script is useful to follow.

> Now continue to relax while I briefly review the ten areas. As I name each part, notice the feelings of relaxation. The first relaxed behavior is Body. Your body is resting comfortably with your spine in a straight line. Head: Your head is aligned with your body and supported by the cushions. Shoulders: Your shoulders are sloped and even. Hands: Your hands are resting on the armrest (your lap) with your fingers slightly curled. Feet: Your feet are resting on the footrest making a "V." Throat: Your throat is smooth and calm. Breathing: Your breathing is slow and regular. Quiet: You are relaxing calmly and quietly. Mouth: Your lips and teeth are parted as your jaw drops into the relaxed position. Eyes: your eyelids are gently closed and smooth.

PROFICIENCY TRAINING PROCEDURES

After all ten items have been learned in the acquisition phase, additional training usually is needed to reach criterion on the BRS and to promote relaxed behaviors in other behavior modalities. Proficiency training involves instruction to the participant, systematic observation of relaxed and unrelaxed behaviors, and verbal feedback concerning the participant's behavior. Instructions to observe the feelings and sensations of relaxation also are a part of training.

Instructions

The participant is asked to relax all ten areas. He or she is told to review the ten items and to observe the relaxed feelings in each area. The participant is told that the trainer will observe the relaxed and unrelaxed behaviors and periodically will provide feedback. Here is an example of proficiency instructions that may be used after acquisition is completed.

> For the next twenty minutes, I would like you to relax all ten of the areas that we have covered. Just to review, please give me the names of the ten areas. [Reinforce correct recitation and provide corrective feedback for any omissions or other errors.] While you are relaxing, I would like you to silently review each of the ten areas and to pay attention to your posture and the sensations of each one. I will periodically observe your relaxation, and if I notice any areas that appear unrelaxed, I will say the name of those areas. For example, if I notice that your breathing is rapid or irregular and that one shoulder is higher than the other, I will say, "breathing [pause] shoulders." You should then pay special attention to the named areas and relax them more. Do not be concerned if you feel the need to move, like if you need to scratch an itch or swallow. Just do what you have to and then return to the relaxed position. For the last few minutes of the session, I will ask you to just continue relaxing on your own but I will not provide any instructions or feedback. Do you have any questions? [Answer questions.] Fine. Now please sit back in the chair and relax all ten parts of your body.

The Observation System

During proficiency training, the trainer systematically observes the participant's behavior to provide feedback. A two-minute interval observation program is recommended. This is frequent enough to prevent faulty habits from developing but not so frequent as to be intrusive. This program is similar to the observational system for relaxation assessment described in Chapter 3, but allows one minute to elapse between each observation interval.

Using the BRS Score Sheet, the trainer first counts the breathing rate for thirty seconds and then observes the other nine behaviors for fifteen seconds. The trainer provides feedback by reporting aloud the one-word label for any item noted to be unrelaxed during the observation period. If all items are relaxed, then the trainer should give descriptive praise. After one minute passes with no observation or feedback, the process is repeated. If a denser schedule of feedback and reinforcement is desired, then observation and feedback can be provided every minute. Alternatively, a leaner schedule can be programmed by allowing more time to elapse between observation periods.

Feedback and Reinforcement

The simplest feedback is to report the one-word label of any behavior observed to be unrelaxed. The participant is instructed to attend to that particular area and relax it. If use of the one-word label is not sufficient to prompt the participant to correct an unrelaxed area, then corrective feedback can be employed. As in the acquisition phase, corrective feedback is a brief description of what the participant is to do to meet the criterion for a particular behavior. Manual guidance usually is not employed during proficiency training. If a particular item is persistently unrelaxed, then more acquisition training may be given prior to the next proficiency session.

If all ten items are relaxed, then the trainer should provide descriptive praise such as "Good, you are doing very well. Your hands are in the curled position." Descriptive praise is contingent on observing the relaxed behaviors and can vary from interval to interval, though all relaxed behaviors should be reinforced over the observation period. Some participants respond better to positive feedback, and it should be included with the corrective feedback even though all ten items are not relaxed. For example, a participant may be told "Your breathing is nice and slow and even, but lower your left shoulder a bit."

An additional feedback procedure that is useful with some people involves showing the participant his or her BRS score from the post training observation period at the conclusion of the session.[6] This score can be calculated easily and quickly (the total number of relaxed behaviors times two gives the percentage relaxed for a five-minute observation period). It can be verbalized as a numerical percentage, or it can be plotted on a graph to show progress over successive sessions. Care should be taken that this does not result in a competitive orientation by the participant. Some participants might want to know how they compare to other people or become concerned about "beating" their previous "scores."

After the first proficiency session, the trainer should ask the participant for their reaction to the feedback. Was it frequent enough, or was it so frequent as to be intrusive? Was it helpful, or was it seen as criticism? The primary criterion for effective feedback is behavior change. The percentage of relaxed behaviors should increase and be maintained at a high level during the post training observation period. BRS scores of 90 percent or better typically are achieved within the first three training sessions. If this is not obtained, then the trainer may want to reevaluate the feedback procedure.

Directing the Participant's Observational Behavior

An important component of relaxation, as discussed in Chapter 2, is observational behavior. Along with instructions for motoric (relaxed posture) and visceral (breathing) behavior, the trainer should provide instructions to guide the participant's observational behavior. The participant observes both overt and covert events. The participant observes (listens to) the trainer's voice providing feedback and is mindful of his or her own posture. But whereas the trainer observes the participant's behavior visually, the participant observes the kinesthetic and proprioceptive events that occur as they relax. In this way, correspondence between public and private events is taught. The trainer also may direct attention to other private events but has no independent means of verifying their occurrence.

A suggestion to observe one or two of the following events should be given every other minute in alternation with relaxation feedback. First are the public events associated with the relaxed behaviors. Participants can be asked to notice their smooth eyelids, parted lips, sloped shoulders, straight alignment of head and torso, curled fingers, and V angle of their feet. Another set of events relates to feelings of heaviness in parts of the body and feelings of support provided by the chair. Participants can be asked to observe the weight of their heads, torsos, arms, hands, and legs resting against the chair. They can be asked to attend to the feelings of support where their heads, shoulders, arms, buttocks, and legs come in contact with the chair. They also can be asked to observe the stimuli of the chair such as the softness of the cushion beneath their head and the smoothness of the surface beneath their fingers.

The stimuli associated with breathing also are useful for directing observational behavior. Participants can be instructed to notice how tension in the chest and shoulders increases slightly as they inhale and tension decreases as they exhale. The temperatures differences between cool air as it is inhaled and warm air as it is exhaled also can be observed. See the later section on *focused breathing*.

Concluding a Session

After 15 or 20 minutes of proficiency training, the trainer should say quietly, "Just continue to relax on your own until you hear the sound of my voice once again." At this point, the BRS is scored for a five-minute observation period, as described in Chapter 3, during which time no feedback or other comments are provided. The BRS score may be quickly calculated and provided to the participant at the end of the session.

At the conclusion of the observation period, the trainer should slowly arouse the participant by saying very quietly, "I am going to count to three. When I say three, slowly open your eyes." A pause of one second should occur between each count. When the participant is alert, the trainer should inquire as to the events observed by the participant. Which events were salient and which were not? Were any observations particularly calming, and were any upsetting? (For example, one woman associated a suggestion of "heaviness in the legs" with concerns about being overweight—not a very calming observation.) In this way, an individualized list of relaxing observational behaviors can be constructed for each participant and used in subsequent sessions.

Summary of Proficiency Training

A proficiency training session comprises several elements. The trainer should first make sure that the participant understands the feedback system and answer any questions. The participant is asked to relax the ten items that have been trained in the acquisition phase. The trainer systematically observes the behaviors listed on the BRS for a one-minute period and provides feedback at the end of each interval. Feedback may be in the form of the one-word label assigned to an unrelaxed behavior, a brief description of how to correct an unrelaxed behavior, or a positive statement noting the participant's success. During alternate minutes, the trainer should direct the participant's observational behavior to the sensations of relaxation such as feelings of heaviness, support, calmness, and peace. After 15 or 20 minutes of training, a five-minute BRS scoring period is conducted, and then the participant is slowly aroused. At the conclusion of each session, the trainer should inquire into the events observed by the participant. A summary BRS score also may be provided to the participant.

Maintenance and Generalization of Relaxation Skills

Relaxation requires practice if the participant is to become proficient in the skill and reap the benefits of training. BRT is similar to other training procedures in this respect. There is consistent evidence that continued practice after the training regimen is an important factor in maintaining the long-term treatment effects.[7,8]

Home Practice and *In Vivo* Use

The importance of home practice should be emphasized. The trainer should discuss with the participant how to incorporate BRT practice time into their daily routine, and how to problem-solve schedule changes so that at least one 20-minute practice session is conducted per day.

Participants often assume that home practice is sufficient to manage their stress, anxiety or discomfort, though often their home is not the context within which the replacement behavior (relaxation) needs to occur. Reviewing homework each session and the data on the *in vivo* use of relaxation allows continuous function-based behavioral assessment leading to the identification of antecedents and consequences for rule-following (pliance),[4] discriminative stimuli for the performance of relaxation, and those that set the occasion for the problem behavior. It is common for participants to report having difficulty relaxing *in vivo* due to the social or physical context. Collaboratively, the trainer and participant can work to identify physical locations that would allow performance of a full or a mini-BRT session. The considerations presented earlier in this chapter concerning the relaxation setting apply to both the home and work environments. For example, Sarah suffered from extreme anxiety following flu-induced panic and vomiting in an underground train filled with passengers. Her anxiety generalized to other settings, including her work, and was especially intense prior to and during staff meetings. Through ongoing function-based assessment, antecedents to her avoidance of performing relaxation were identified—her work space was too observable by her supervisor, and she reported concern about punishment for "doing nothing." It was agreed that both long-duration and mini-BRT relaxation sessions could occur throughout the day by taking scheduled bathroom breaks, where she could use the private rest room and relax in the upright position while seated on the toilet. She agreed that a mini-BRT relaxation session in the rest room could be carried out immediately prior to a staff meeting, as well as in the meeting itself. Her place of employment also had lounge chairs in a foyer that looked out upon a garden. She agreed that she would practice long-duration relaxation after each lunch break using the foyer chairs.

The home practice form (Appendix A) provides a prompt for the participant to practice BRT. The record of the number of occurrences of practice and self-reported levels of relaxation provides feedback to the trainer on issues that may need to be addressed. Another variation that is clinically useful is the Pre-Post Relaxation and Distress Rating Form. (Appendix E).

Contracting for Maintenance

Planned action is needed to ensure that the gains made through BRT generalize and are maintained in other settings. As an antecedent control procedure, contingency contracts encompass the manipulation of self-generated plys, social reinforcement for pliance, and naturally occurring reinforcers for engaging in relaxation (the desired alternative behavior). Relapse prevention contracts have a long history and empirical support for their use as a maintenance intervention is equally widespread and ranges from organizational behavior management to addictions.[9-11]

A general model for contracting for maintenance is described below. Contracts can be modified to promote the maintenance of relaxation skills among children, adolescents, and individuals with disabilities.[12,13] Discussion of maintaining progress based on BRT commences three to four weeks prior to the last session. Conversation about maintenance and preventing relapse is based on the data, both acquisition and *in vivo* recording of distress or other problem behaviors. The first conversation is general and brief: for example, "You are doing very well managing the stress in your life. Let's talk about how you can maintain this success." Two weeks prior to the end of formal delivery of services, further conversation related to maintenance is linked to the participant's values for living and their treatment goal. The use of a maintenance contract is introduced as a means to make a public commitment to continue to use and practice relaxation skills. (See Appendix F). The participant is given the contract and asked to review it at home. At the last session the contract is reviewed, questions addressed, and it is signed by both parties.

For the first two weeks of the six-week post-intervention period, the trainer initiates brief weekly telephone contact with the participant to provide social reinforcement and problem-solve challenges to maintenance of behavior change. Each week for the next six weeks, the participant sends the completed homework to the trainer. At the end of the week six, the scheduled follow up assessment occurs and appropriate indirect assessment occurs along with direct assessment of relaxed behavior. Further follow up is scheduled as needed.

VARIATIONS OF STANDARD BRT

It is usually helpful to supplement fully reclined BRT to promote transfer to home and work situations that enhance relaxation effects. These additions allow the participant to engage in relaxed behaviors throughout the day in situations that do not allow a recumbent position. They are, in effect, partial relaxation procedures and not intended to serve as substitutes for full practice. They help to strengthen the participant's discrimination of arousing events and provide calming alternative responses in those situations.

Two variations, *upright relaxation* and *mini-relaxation*, are particularly useful. In addition, *focused breathing* is a technique that is helpful in everyday arousing situations. But these should not take the place of the daily relaxation period.

Upright Relaxation Training (UBRT)

An important aspect of relaxation is that it be portable. A central theme of this book is that relaxation is a skill to be employed in a variety of arousing settings. Reclining chairs are not commonly available in most environments, nor is it possible to stretch out in full relaxed postures at work, at social gatherings, or while commuting. To enhance the transfer of relaxation to a wide variety of environments, a participant may be taught to relax while seated in an upright position. Such opportunities are widely available—in offices, homes, waiting rooms, cars, and buses—offering ubiquitous opportunities to relax.

A study by Krmpotich[14] measured tension levels of several major muscle groups in six adults (three males and three females) as they assumed various postures while seated in an upright chair. From this and other research[15] we have devised an Upright Behavioral Relaxation Scale (UBRS) defining postures requiring the least muscle tension to sustain while seated in an upright position.

After participants have reached proficiency in relaxing while reclined, it is a simple matter to teach them the behaviors on the UBRS. The same procedures of modeling, prompting, and performance feedback employed in teaching the reclined behaviors are applicable in teaching the upright postures as well.

The ten upright relaxed behaviors are as follows:

1. *Back.*

    RELAXED. The spine is perpendicular to the floor with the shoulder blades and the buttocks touching the back of the chair. A slight lordosis (concave lower back) is recommended. (See Photo 4.1A).

    UNRELAXED. Any of the following are observed: (a) bent forward so that shoulders are not in contact with chair back (Photo 4.1B); (b) leaning back so

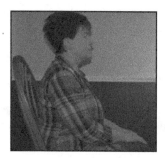

Photo 4.1A

that buttocks are not in contact with the chair back (Photo 4.1C); (c) leaning to one side so that the spine is not perpendicular (Photo 4.1D).

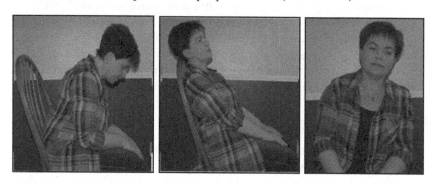

Photos 4.1B, C, and D

2. *Head.*

RELAXED. The head is upright and motionless with the nose in midline with the body. A useful metaphor is to picture the head as a ball balanced on a stick (the spine). (See Photo 4.2A)

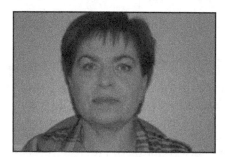

Photo 4.2A

UNRELAXED. The head is tilted forward (Photo 4.2B), backward (Photo 4.2C), or to one side (Photo 4.2D).

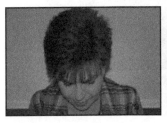 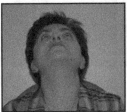 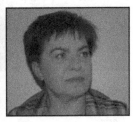

Photos 4.2B, C, and D

3. *Arms.*

RELAXED. Arms are bent approximately 120 degrees at the elbow with the wrists resting on the thigh, approximately halfway between the hip and the knee. These dimensions may vary depending on the participant's body proportions. Proper placement of the arms ensures that the shoulders are even. (Photo 4.3A)

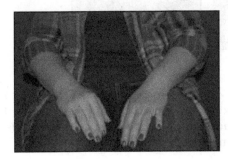

Photo 4.3A

UNRELAXED. Any of the following are observed: (a) arms akimbo (Photo 4.3B); (b) leaning forward on arms (Photo 4.3C); (c) arms hanging at sides (Photo 4.3D); (d) movement of arms.

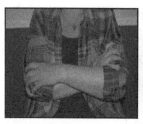 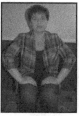 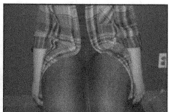

Photos 4.3B, C, and D

4. *Legs.*

   RELAXED. Legs straight and feet flat on the floor with approximately 90 degree angle at the knees and ankles. (Photo 4.4A, B).

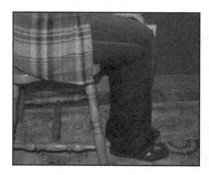 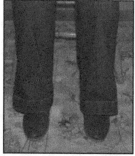

Photos 4.4A and B

   UNRELAXED. Any of the following are observed: (a) legs crossed at knee or ankle (Photo 4.4C); (b) legs extended so that knee angle is greater than 90 degrees (Photo 4.4D) or legs tucked under chair so that knee angle is less than 90 degrees (Photo 4.4E); (c) movement of legs or feet.

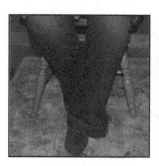 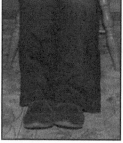 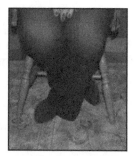

Photos 4.4C, D, and E

The BRS Score Sheet may be used in the training and scoring of upright BRT with two changes: "back" substituted for "body" and "arms" substituted for "shoulders." The following items are the same as defined on the reclined BRS: *Eyes, Mouth, Throat, Hands, Quiet,* and *Breathing*.

Mini-BRT Relaxation

As the participant becomes proficient in relaxing in the reclining chair as evidenced by BRS scores, self-ratings, the Tension Self-Rating Form (Appendix A), and other measures, they can be introduced to the practice of mini-BRT relaxation. In essence, this involves relaxing parts of the body while engaging in other activities. It is similar in concept to Jacobson's "differential relaxation." Daily activities that occur routinely should be reviewed with the participant to determine how and where he or she can employ mini-relaxation. Rehearsal and role-playing of mini-relaxation in various situations can be incorporated into the training session. Any of the behaviors defined on the BRS or UBRS may be relaxed in the everyday environment, depending on other activities of the person. For example, mouth and throat can be relaxed in nonsocial situations in which the participant does not have to speak or be concerned with their mouth hanging open. Breathing can be relaxed in situations not requiring speech or exertion. Hands can be relaxed in situations in which they are not required for manipulation. Shoulders and back should be relaxed while engaged in seated activities such as driving, typing, or other desk work.

When a person is very actively engaged in a task, they should be encouraged to take periodic mini-relaxation breaks to literally "catch their breath" by closing the eyes, breathing slowly and evenly, opening the mouth, lowering the shoulders, and curling the fingers. Such breaks may last from a few seconds to a few minutes in duration.

The trainer should point out that the participant can use regularly occurring environmental events as reminders to engage in mini-relaxation. Events such as hanging up the telephone after a call, completing a section of a book or newspaper, or stopping at a red light while driving, can serve as mini-relaxation cues. For very busy people, a small dot of white typing correction fluid placed on the wristwatch crystal serves as a helpful prompt to take a mini-relaxation break.

FOCUSED BREATHING

Breathing is visceral behavior that occurs naturally and regularly for most people most of the time. Many relaxation procedures, including BRT, PMR, and various meditation methods, ask the participant to attend to, and perhaps alter, some aspect of their breathing. Thus breathing is, to some extent, an operant response under control of contingencies such as verbal instructions.

The following is a list of breathing maneuvers characteristic of many relaxation and meditation training procedures:[16-18]

1. **Observation of breathing**, in which the person is instructed, or instructs themselves, to concentrate on specified aspects of breathing.
2. **Nasal breathing**, in which air is inhaled and exhaled through the nose rather than the mouth.
3. **Regular breathing**, in which the rate and magnitude of inhale-exhale cycles is consistent over time.
4. **Slow breathing**, in which the rate is decreased from the uninstructed frequency.
5. **Abdominal breathing**, in which the abdomen rises with each inhalation and falls during exhalation, while the upper chest remains relatively still.

BRT involves Items 1 through 4 of this list, although only rate of breathing and gross disruptions, such as coughing, are objectively observed and scored on the BRS. *Focused breathing* involves including the fifth item, abdominal breathing, as well as the first four.

Abdominal breathing is also termed *diaphragmatic* breathing, because it emphasizes use of the diaphragm, the band of muscles between the lungs and the stomach. Inhalation occurs when the chest volume expands, thus drawing air into the lungs, and exhalation occurs when chest volume decreases, forcing air out. The diaphragm is much more efficient than chest and shoulder muscles in controlling chest volume, and allows those muscles to remain relaxed while breathing. Diaphragmatic breathing may have widespread effects on other visceral responses, particularly vasomotor activity, with growing support for its benefit.[19-22] Diaphragmatic breathing has been found to be effective for asthma, motion sickness, migraine headache, cardiac disorders, and hyperventilation. Fried[21] proposed that "hypoxia" was a key feature of many stress disorders that could be remedied by diaphragmatic breathing.

Training in focused breathing should begin only after proficiency has been achieved with BRT. Because participants may achieve 90 percent or better relaxed behaviors on the BRS within as few as two sessions, focused breathing may be incorporated into the BRT procedure very early for some participants.

Rationale for Focused Breathing

Focused breathing can be presented as an enhancement of relaxation that has specific effects on the problem for which the participant is seeking treatment. While the literature on diaphragmatic breathing is growing, the trainer should not overstate its benefits. An evidence-based approach is advised. A statement to the following effect creates a positive but not unrealistic expectancy.

> Focused breathing is based on methods that have been practiced for thousands of years for achieving calmness and reduction of tension. It involves learning to use the diaphragm, the band of muscles between the lungs and the stomach, to draw air into the lungs. Focused breathing is more efficient, allowing you to relax your neck and shoulder muscles while breathing. [This may be helpful for tension-related disorders such as headache and myofacial pain dysfunction.] Focused breathing may result in relaxation in the vascular system and is helpful for vascular disorders such as migraine.[19] It is incompatible with rapid, shallow breathing such as occurs in asthma.[20] Focusing one's attention on slow rhythmic breathing can have a general calming effect that is helpful for anxiety disorders [21,22]

Training Procedures

Precise measurement of diaphragmatic and thoracic activity during breathing requires pneumographic or electronic strain-gauge equipment, which is beyond the means of most clinicians. Fortunately, it is possible for the participant to place their hands so that both the participant and the trainer can observe the relative motion of the chest and abdomen. The following procedure has been found to be consistent with measures provided by pneumographic recording.[16]

While reclined in a relaxed posture, the participant is instructed using the following steps.

> **HAND PLACEMENT.** Place your right hand on your stomach, between the bottom of your rib cage and your navel. [For most people, this is just above their belt lines.] Place your left hand on your chest, on your breast bone (sternum) just below your collar bone (clavicle).
>
> **BASELINE BREATHING.** Now just breathe regularly through your nose and notice the rise and fall of your hands as you breathe in (inhale)

and breathe out (exhale). [Observe the participant and point out the occurrence of diaphragmatic or chest (thoracic) breathing.]

ABDOMINAL PRACTICE. As you breathe in (inhale), imagine your stomach to be a balloon that inflates, lifting your right hand. As you breathe out (exhale), the balloon deflates and your right hand falls. Your left hand remains still as your right hand rises and falls.

FEEDBACK. Do not try to force it. Just attend to the motion of your hands and the feelings in your chest. Allow your right hand to rise and fall while your left hand remains still.

Some people find additional imagery to be helpful. The participant can be instructed to imagine that his or her right hand is a boat, rising and falling on the slow, rolling waves of the ocean, while the left hand sits quietly at the dock.

The trainer should observe the motion of the participant's hands for several breathing cycles. Some people are able to achieve the described pattern very quickly, whereas others have difficulty. Most are able to increase the amplitude of abdominal breathing, as shown by the motion of the right hand, but continue to breathe thoracically as well. If this is the case, then the trainer should comment approvingly on the abdominal changes but should not strongly disapprove of the thoracic component, only mentioning to keep the left hand still. A shaping process should be employed in which approval is given for one aspect of the breathing pattern and, with practice, the other aspect declines. The participant may attempt to breathe deeply by raising and lowering his or her shoulders. The trainer should point this out and instruct the participant to keep their shoulders still.

SLOW BREATHING. Next, slow your breathing by pausing very briefly at the top and bottom of each breath, just a half second or so. Do not hold your breath or pause so that you are uncomfortable.

ADDITIONAL PRACTICE AND FEEDBACK. The trainer should continue to praise positive aspects of the breathing pattern, with occasional corrective feedback for negative aspects.

TENSION RELEASE. Notice how there is a slight increase in tension as you breathe in and a decrease as you breathe out. Concentrate on the tension flowing out with each breath. Feel a slight increase in tension as you inhale, and then let go as you exhale. Each time you exhale, feel the tension leaving your body.

Focused Breathing in Combination with BRT

What follows is a script to use when combing focused breathing and BRT.

> Now we are going to practice the abdominal breathing and the relaxed postures together. Silently review the relaxed postures to yourself, but leave your hands on your chest and abdomen. Also notice the motion of your hands, the slight pauses in your breathing, and the release of tension each time you exhale.

Provide BRS feedback along with the breathing feedback at two-minute intervals, as described earlier, for 10 to 15 minutes. By placing the hands in this fashion, the criteria for hands and shoulders on the BRS may be disrupted; this should be disregarded for feedback and BRS scoring.

PLACEMENT OF HANDS AT SIDES. After one or two sessions with the participant's hands on the chest and abdomen, the trainer may say:

> This time, I would like you to place your hands on the arms of the chair. Continue to breathe with your abdomen rising and falling and your chest remaining still. Notice the sensations in your chest and abdomen as you breathe and let go of all tension as you exhale.

There may be some disruption of diaphragmatic breathing when the hand placement no longer provides feedback, but this usually is transitory.

Some Difficulties with Focused Breathing

Participants sometimes report unease when they first try abdominal breathing. It is foreign to their usual breathing patterns, and the awareness of and attempt to control a behavior that usually is automatic can be disconcerting. These facts should be pointed out to those who express difficulty, reassuring them that their experience is not unusual. Like any new skill, such as riding a bicycle or swimming, there is often an initial period of awareness of awkwardness. But by consistent practice, most people can learn to become proficient and comfortable with this new style of breathing. Reassurance, encouragement, and positive feedback are sufficient to deal with problems.

In some cases, it may be helpful to take more time on each of the steps outlined above rather than trying to accomplish all of them in one or two sessions. Also, it may be helpful to provide additional BRT proficiency sessions before introducing focused breathing. When making the transition from hands on the stomach and chest to hands off, it often is helpful to allow the participant to continue to use one hand on either the chest or the abdomen, in alternating fashion, while placing the other at his or her side. The trainer should be careful not to blame the participant for their difficulty and should take responsibility for the pace of training.

USING FOCUSED BREATHING. Participants should be instructed to make focused breathing an integral part of their BRT home practice. It can be incorporated with Upright as well as Reclined BRT, and be included in their mini-relaxation routine. In fact, it can be used by itself as a "breather," taking less than a minute, to calm them self in the midst of a hectic situation.

ISSUES THAT MAY INTERFERE WITH BRT. For most participants, BRT proceeds in a straightforward fashion. Some, however, experience problems that require special attention. These include difficulties with particular postures, falling asleep, wandering thoughts, an aversion to being observed, and a variety of phenomena sometimes referred to as *relaxation-induced anxiety* or RIA. These events are described below, along with some suggestions on how to deal with them.

DIFFICULTIES WITH INDIVIDUAL RELAXED POSTURES

Certain items seem to give rise to problems that, while not frequent, occur often enough to merit some consideration on how to deal with them.

BODY. Placement of the torso in the recliner provides the foundation for all the rest of the relaxed behaviors. It is important that the participant sits all the way back in the chair so that their lower back is supported when reclined. If the buttocks are scooted forward, low back discomfort may occur due to lack of support. Be sure to instruct the participant right off to "sit all the way back" and to check that they do so.

SHOULDERS. The position of the participant's hands on the armrest affects the extent to which the shoulders are raised or lowered. Hands placed too far up the armrest may produce a shrugged posture in the shoulders, and too far down may stretch the shoulder muscles, in both instances resulting in excess tension. In some cases, a participant may report shoulder discomfort. It may be helpful to ask the participant to focus on the tension in their trapezius muscles, which, with permission, the trainer can indicate with a gentle touch. Then ask that they slide their hands slowly up and down the armrest, to determine the point at which least tension is experienced. Note that the hands should remain in the relaxed, claw-like posture.

HEAD. Many people habitually carry their head tilted to one side or the other. Consequently, when their head is placed in the relaxed, mid-line posture, some may feel this to be "crooked" or uncomfortable. Usually an explanation of the commonly occurring asymmetric posture, and reassurance that, with practice, the relaxed position will come to feel natural, is sufficient to address their concerns.

MOUTH. From childhood on, people are commonly taught that it is impolite to have their mouth open in public. Thus the dropped jaw, with lips and teeth slightly parted, may not feel acceptable for some folks. Again, reassurance that this posture reduces facial tension and will, with practice, feel natural and comfortable, is an acceptable answer. Participants may need to be reminded to breathe through their nose even while their mouth is open.

SLEEP. Participants have been known to fall asleep during BRT. The difference between relaxation and sleep may not be immediately apparent to the observer, but there are some tell-tale clues to watch for. The participant's head may loll to one side or snoring may commence. During training, the person may not be responsive to corrective feedback given by the trainer. During an observation period, when no feedback is provided, the trainer should mark on the BRS score sheet the point at which sleep behavior is suspected.

To awaken a participant, call their name softly, e.g., "Dana, are you sleeping?" then repeat a bit louder if there is no response. If still no reaction, gently touch their forearm while saying their name. When awake, tell the participant, "You became so relaxed that you fell asleep. That is not a bad thing, but there is a difference between sleep and relaxation and we want to work on relaxation skills." In other words, provide reassurance but focus on the task at hand.

In other instances, a participant may exhibit a startle reaction and suddenly jerk awake, in what is termed a myoclonic or hypnogogic jerk.[23] This may be accompanied by signs of sympathetic arousal, such as rapid heart rate and hyperventilation. The participant should be assured that this is a benign event that some people experience in early stages of sleep. Ask if the participant has had this happen in their home environment. While there is speculation that hypnogogic phenomena are related to stress, or caffeine, or irregular sleep schedules, there is no systematic research pinpointing a cause.

Participants may also report falling asleep during their home relaxation practice. Wherever it happens, if sleep intrudes on relaxation, then the participant's sleep schedule should be discussed. This could provide an avenue into areas of stress that affect their sleep. If insomnia is a problem, relaxation may be helpful as part of a sleep hygiene program. But this should not take the place of waking relaxation practice and implementation in daily life.

Sleep apnea is a rare occurrence. It is characterized by a period of no respiration, neither inhalation or exhalation, perhaps lasting a minute or more, followed by gasping or snorting as breathing resumes. Typically, the person does not awaken as they would from a myoclonic jerk. For example, if the rate on the thirty-second breathing observation period on the BRS is scored as one or zero, the participant's respiration should be closely observed. If apnea is suspected, the participant should be awakened and the matter discussed further. This is not a benign condition and the participant should be encouraged to consult their physician.

WANDERING THOUGHTS. Sometimes a participant may report that, as they relaxed, "their mind started to wander." In behavioral terms, they were attending to covert verbal or observational stimuli other than the proprioceptive or kinesthetic stimuli that occur as a function of relaxation. Or perhaps external environmental stimuli intruded. Because of the "problem of privacy,"[12] special efforts must be made to gain instructional control over relaxation-related observational behaviors.

Several steps may be useful in increasing the likelihood that the participant's observational behavior is under stimulus control of the relevant events. First, inquiry is necessary. After the final observation period of a training session, or in reviewing home practice, it is useful to ask what the person noticed, what they felt or thought about, as they relaxed. They may report thinking about unfinished tasks, upcoming meetings, or previous interactions with various people. The trainer should accept this as "normal," but a possible hindrance in gaining the full benefits of relaxation. The next step is to provide a rationale for attending to relaxation-relevant stimuli, such as linking them to the goals of treatment or the "values for living" established in initial assessments (Chapter 3). The following step is to identify the discursive thoughts (e.g., wondering what to make for dinner) and use it as a cue for attending to some covert event related to relaxation (e.g., feeling the softness of the cushion behind one's head). It might be helpful to provide a refresher on some of these private stimuli (see preceding section on *Directing the Participant's Observational Behavior*). Finally, feedback and social reinforcement should be provided contingent on maintenance of the overt relaxed behaviors and for verbal report of attending to relaxation-relevant stimuli.

Complaints about Observation or Feedback

An occasional participant may express discomfort with being watched during the observation period. It is appropriate to discuss the participant's feelings and provide reassurance. Perhaps the discomfort is a reaction to a novel situation and will fade with continued training. Inquiry into the participant's covert observational and verbal behavior may be indicated. What are they attending to and talking to themselves about? Redirection of their observational behavior to the proprioceptive and kinesthetic feelings of relaxed postures, as described above, is helpful in this regard.

A related issue is that a participant may report feeling "pressured" into performing better, and perceive feedback about unrelaxed postures as criticism. Again, discussion and reassurance can clarify that just about all learning of new skills requires trial and error. Feedback is constructive when it helps to learn from one's mistakes. Also, providing positive feedback for correctly performed behaviors may make training feel less aversive.

Relaxation-Induced Anxiety

"Relaxation-induced anxiety" (RIA) references a broad class of unpleasant reactions some participants experience during relaxation training. It can be measured by various self-report anxiety questionnaires as well as a specific Response to Relaxation Session rating scale.[24] RIA has been observed in treatment research programs that include a variety of training methods, including progressive muscle relaxation, mantra meditation, EMG biofeedback, slowed diaphragmatic breathing, and calming imagery.

Inasmuch as clinical research involves systematic comparison of two or more treatment packages in which strict protocols are adhered to, RIA is regarded as an uncontrolled variable that can be analyzed post hoc to see how it impacts treatment outcome. For example, persons meeting diagnostic criteria for Generalized Anxiety Disorder, who are thought to be particularly prone to RIA, received two differing cognitive-behavioral treatment programs, both of which included relaxation training. Overall, both groups achieved significant improvements on a variety of clinical measures regardless of RIA scores during treatment. A finer-grain analysis showed that lower levels of RIA during the last phase of treatment was associated with better scores on some measures.[25]

Thus, even in rigorous research programs, RIA does not seem to be a major impediment. In clinical settings with individual participants, there is usually room for improvisation and the participant's reactions can be addressed on a personal basis. Rather than a vague notion of anxiety, it is best to determine what the participant is experiencing across the four response modalities. Is it verbal, as in covert self-talk (e.g., "I can't do this. This is pointless. I'm giving up control"); visceral (e.g., heart pounding, shortness of breath, cold hands); motor (e.g., trembling, tight feeling in shoulders); or observational (e.g., attending to motor or visceral sensations, feeling dizzy)? Often, just acknowledging and accepting bumps in the road decreases their potency in impeding progress. In other cases, a sub-routine may be necessary to address the issue, such as alternatives to negative self-talk or tense-release exercises, *a la* Jacobson, for recalcitrant muscle groups.

MODIFICATIONS OF THE BRT PROTOCOL FOR DIVERSE POPULATIONS AND INDIVIDUAL NEEDS

All relaxation training procedures are adjusted to meet the needs of individual participants. Even the most standardized procedures, such as Bernstein and Borkovec's[26] version of PMR, are modified for particular clinical or research protocols. This practice allows better outcomes for a particular individual or group. However, in the long run, unless the modifications are carefully documented, this practice adds little to our knowledge base of which procedures work best in which circumstances and for which participants. Each of the elements of BRT, described above, is subject to modification so as to better accommodate special needs. These elements include the setting, the rationale, the procedure itself, the use of consequences, and maintenance procedures.

Antecedents of Training

SETTING. The setting for BRT with participants with unique challenges should follow the guidelines described earlier with respect to minimizing distractions. It may be helpful to acclimate the participant to the training room for a few sessions prior to commencing BRT, perhaps by using it as a place for review of various aspects of the participant's program or just for "small talk."

ORGANIZATION OF TRAINING SESSIONS. Care should be taken that the scheduled training time does not interfere with some favored activity of the participant. Initial sessions should be scheduled at least once a day if at all possible. As acquisition occurs, sessions can be spaced out to two or three times weekly. The general training sequence outlined above should be followed, but session duration should be shorter, especially early in training.

RATIONALE. The participant should be given an explanation for relaxation training according to their level of understanding. The purpose of training should be related to an area of benefit for the participant, such as

"This can help you control your temper," or simply "This can help you feel better." Undue expectations should not be encouraged, but the idea of practice and improvement should be fostered. For example, a participant may be told, "Relaxation won't make your headaches stop right away, but if you do this every day, they won't be so bad." People should not be summarily assigned to treatment but rather should be allowed to choose whether or not to participate.

Training Procedures

ACQUISITION TRAINING. The four steps described earlier—*labeling, modeling, imitation,* and *feedback*—are employed for each of the ten behaviors on the BRS. However, the entire process may be slowed for persons with special needs, with deliberate shaping of increasing durations and chaining of successive behaviors. Extrinsic consequences, such as tokens or preferred activities/events, may be added to the usual social praise. It is especially helpful to begin training with those behaviors that already were relaxed during baseline so that the participant can start off successfully. A general strategy is to identify, label, and model the first item and request the participant to imitate it for successive durations of 15, 30, and 60 seconds. The second behavior is trained in a similar fashion for 15, 30, and 60 seconds. The participant is then asked to demonstrate both behaviors together for a 60-second period. The third behavior is then trained and imitated for 15, 30, and 60 seconds, and then all three are displayed for 60 seconds. In some cases, especially early in training for people who have difficulty even sitting still, we have found it helpful to count the seconds aloud. Also, the initial time requirements may be shortened for some participants to as little as five seconds. This process continues until all ten items have been trained. Corrective verbal feedback is provided immediately, contingent on any unrelaxed behavior occurring for an already trained item. The participant is allowed two seconds to self-correct, and then further instruction or manual guidance is employed as appropriate. Praise is given on successful completion of each temporal criterion. Typically, one to three items can be trained in each session. Each session starts with the participant being told the labels of all behaviors trained up to that point and being asked to demonstrate all of them together for 60 seconds. Retraining of behaviors that do not meet the criterion should be done prior to proceeding with new ones.

EXTRINSIC CONSEQUENCES. Token reinforcers, such as poker chips or coins, may be helpful for some participants. This system can be part of an ongoing program in the training facility or can be set up especially for BRT.

The details of the program should be worked out with the participant and their parents or staff prior to training. Delivery of tokens should be concurrent with praise for meeting a behavioral criterion. Tokens can be dropped into a jar or can, making a clinking sound, so that the participant does not have to watch for token delivery. Tokens also may be taken away for disruptive behavior during the session. Tokens should be exchanged for backup reinforcers immediately after the conclusion of the session. Extrinsic reinforcers such as soda, candy bars, or excursions also may be awarded after a session for compliance during the session. Using immediate reinforcers helps the special needs participant stay motivated so that the long-term gains of relaxation can accrue.

PROFICIENCY TRAINING. After all ten behaviors are acquired, the proficiency training procedure, described earlier, is employed with a few modifications. The duration of the training session may be shortened to ten or fifteen minutes. Corrective feedback rather than the one-word label often is necessary, and manual guidance may continue to be employed. Positive verbal feedback for relaxed behavior is effective for special populations and should be interspersed frequently during training. If a token or other extrinsic reinforcement system was employed during acquisition, then it is desirable to fade it out during the proficiency phase. If tokens are continued, then they can be awarded at the end of the session on the basis of the BRS score obtained during the assessment period. Even without tokens, we have found graphic feedback in the form of a histogram displaying the current BRS score and previous scores presented after each session along with suitable praise, is a good way to maintain interest and cooperation. The proficiency criterion for special participants may be set lower than that for other people. We have used both 80 percent and 90 percent relaxed behavior on the BRS for two successive sessions, with a minimum of six training sessions. The capabilities of individual participants should be taken into account in setting a criterion, but the trainer should be careful not to underestimate their abilities and to be alert to ways in which to modify the program to improve success.

Maintenance and Generalization with Diverse Populations

As discussed earlier, practice of relaxation skills on their own is critical at times other than training sessions and when feeling distressed or agitated. Higher-functioning individuals can make use of the Tension Self-Rating Scale (Appendix A) to monitor their own practice and progress. Contingency contracting, as discussed above, for practice and use of self-managed relaxation can improve both maintenance and generalization of skills. In structured living facilities, practice times can be incorporated into daily routines, with unobtrusive checks by professional staff and assessed using the Residential BRT Checklist (See Appendix G). For caregivers in home settings, the Caregiver Reclined Relaxed Behavior Rating Form can be used during practice sessions for use of relaxation in times of distress (see Appendix H). Mini-relaxation training often is appropriate for special participants. The goal of BRT for these participants, as for any participants, is for relaxation to be incorporated into their daily lives.

Although persons with a wide variety of disorders can learn relaxation fairly readily, it is equally obvious that they must also receive training in how to utilize these skills in everyday situations. Relaxation may have some general calming effects, but it is not like a tranquilizing medication. Many studies have shown that for relaxation to be truly effective, individuals need to learn the cues in their physical and social environments, and even in their own bodies, that signal it is time to relax.

TRAINING BRT TRAINERS

Individuals who have no experience conducting relaxation training may find it difficult to chain together the complex repertoire required to teach relaxation. Lundervold and colleagues[27] validated an acquisition training protocol, based on the procedures described above, for use in training the trainers. This training protocol is included in Appendix I.

The training procedures were task analyzed to allow systematic assessment and instruction of the trainer. Behavioral skill training (instructions, modeling, behavioral rehearsal, feedback, reinforcement) procedures were used to teach the relaxation training skills. Figure 4.1 depicts the performance of the trainer and the participant who was being taught to relax. Trainers were undergraduate research assistants who had mastered direct observation of relaxed behavior. As can be seen, simply giving the trainer the list of relaxed behaviors and definitions and instructed to "teach the participant to relax" (baseline) was ineffective in improving the performance of the participant.

Training skills for BRT improved significantly following behavioral skills training and use of the BRT acquisition protocol. Similarly, the participant's performance of relaxed behavior also systematically improved. Assessment of generalized training skills was also demonstrated with two new participants.

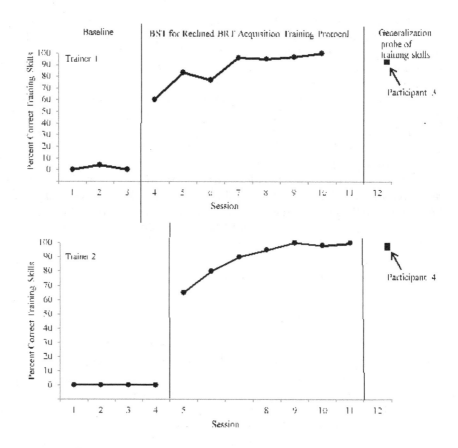

Figure 4.1 Percent correct responses and generalized performance in the use of the Behavioral Relaxation Training Acquisition protocol.

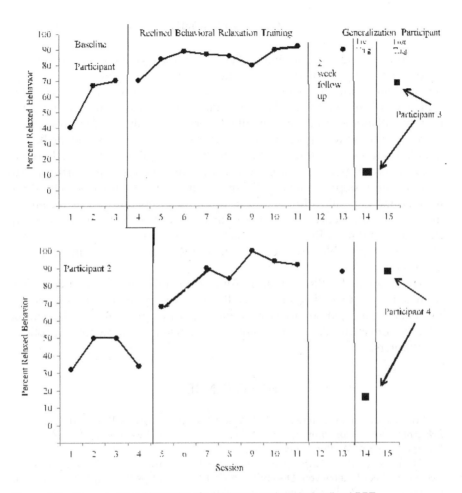

Figure 4.2. Percent relaxed behavior of participants undergoing reclined BRT.

CONCLUSIONS

Behavioral Relaxation Training (BRT) is comprised of ten overt postures or actions that are presented to the participant in sequence by verbal description and modeling. Acquisition proceeds in a cumulative manner, with the trainer providing verbal feedback or manual guidance as needed, until the participant attains proficiency on all ten items, typically within two sessions, or more for those with special needs. Performance is measured on the Behavioral Relaxation Scale (BRS), an interval observational recording method that yields a percent relaxed score. Proficiency training allows the participant to become more adept at relaxing and more attuned to its covert aspects. Maintenance and generalization of relaxation skills are encouraged by a commitment to home practice and by teaching variations in BRT, namely Upright Relaxation and Mini-Relaxation, which promote relaxation in everyday situations. Some possible adverse reactions to BRT and ways of handling them are discussed.

The rationale for BRT is that it provides an antidote for stressful or painful reactions to upsetting situations. It is easily combined with other cognitive-behavioral methods to meet a wide range of problems. It also can be adapted for children and adults with special needs, as shown in the following chapters.

REFERENCES

[1] Main, C., Keefe, F. J., Jensen, M. P., Vlaey, J. W. S., & Vowles, K. E. (2015). *Fordyce's Behavioral methods for chronic pain and illness*. Republished with invited commentary. Philadelphia, PA: Wolters Kluwer Health.

[2] Harris, R. (2008). *Clarifying your values*. (Adapted from Tobias Lundgren's Bull's Eye Worksheet). Retrieved December 5, 2018 from https://thehappinesstrap.com/upimages/Long_Bull%27s_Eye_Worksheet.pdf

[3] Skinner, B. F. (1969). *Contingencies of reinforcement*. NY: Appleton Century Crofts.

[4] Zettle, R., & Hayes, S.C. (1989). Rule-governed behavior: A potential theoretical frame-work for cognitive behavior therapy. In P.C. Kendall (Ed.), *Advances in cognitive-behavioral research and therapy*, Vol. 1 (pp. 77–118). NY: Academic Press.

[5] Wolpe, J. (1958). *Psychotherapy by reciprocal inhibition*. Stanford, CA: Stanford University Press.

[6] Lundervold, D. A., Talley, C., & Buermann, M. (2008). Effect of Behavioral Activation Treatment on chronic fibromyalgia pain: Replication and extension. *International Journal of Behavioral Consultation and Therapy*, 4, 146–157. http://dx.doi.org/10.1037/h0100839

[7] Blanchard, E. B., & Andrasik, F. (1985). *Management of chronic headaches*. NY: Pergamon.

[8]Reinking, R. H., & Hutchings, D. (1981). Follow-up to: Tension headaches: What form of therapy is most effective? *Biofeedback and Self-Regulation, 6,* 57–62. https://doi.org/10.1007/BF00998793

[9]Marlatt, G. A., & Gordon, J. R. (1980). Determinants of relapse: Implications for the maintenance of behavior change. In P. O. Davidson & S. M. Davidson (Eds.), Behavioral medicine: Changing health lifestyles (pp. 410–452). NY: Brunner/Mazel.

[10]Marx, R.D. (1982). Relapse prevention for managerial training: A model for maintenance of behavior change. *Academy of Management Review, 7*(3), 433–441. https://doi.org/10.5465/amr.1982.4285359

[11]Hendershot, C.S., Witkiewitz, K., George, W.H., & Marlatt, G.A. Relapse prevention for addictive behaviors. *Substance Abuse Treatment and Prevention Policy 6, 17 (2011).* https://doi.org/10.1186/1747-597X-6-17. Retrieved on February 7, 2019 from https://substanceabusepolicy.biomedcentral.com/articles/10.1186/1747-597X-6-17.

[12]Mruzek, D. W., Cohen, C., & Smith, T. J. (2007). Contingency contracting with students with autism spectrum disorders in a public school setting. *Journal of Developmental and Physical Disabilities, 19*(2), 103–114. https://doi.org/10.1007/s10882-007-9036-x

[13]Hoelscher, T. J., Lichstein, K. L., & Rosenthal, T. L. (1986). Home relaxation practice in hypertension treatment: Objective assessment and compliance induction. *Journal of Consulting and Clinical Psychology, 54*(2), 217–221. http://dx.doi.org/10.1037/0022-006X.54.2.217

[14]Krmpotich, J. D. (1986). *Behavioral relaxation in an upright chair: An electromyographic analysis.* Unpublished master's thesis, Southern Illinois University at Carbondale.

[15]Poppen, R., Hanson, H., & Ip, S. V. (1988). Generalization of EMG biofeedback training. *Biofeedback and Self-Regulation, 13,* 235–243. doi: 10.1007/BF00999172

[16]Bacon, M., & Poppen, R. (1985). A behavioral analysis of diaphragmatic breathing and its effects on peripheral temperature. *Journal of Behavior Therapy & Experimental Psychiatry,16*(1),15–21. https://doi.org/10.1016/0005-7916(85)90025-4

[17]Boyer, B. A., & Poppen, R. (1995). Effects of abdominal and thoracic breathing upon multiple-site electromyography and peripheral skin temperature. *Perceptual and Motor Skills, 81*(1), 3–14. https://doi.org/10.2466/pms.1995.81.1.3

[18]Fried, R., & Grimaldi, J. (1993). *The psychology and physiology of breathing.* NY: Plenum Press. http://dx.doi.org/10.1007/978-1-4899-1239-8.

[19]Kaushik, R., Kaushik, R. M., Mahajan, S. K., & Rajesh, V. (2005). Biofeedback assisted diaphragmatic breathing and systematic relaxation versus propranolol in long term prophylaxis of migraine. *Complementary Therapy and Medicine, 13*(3), 165–74. https://doi.org/10.1016/j.ctim.2005.04.004

[20]Peper, E., & Tibbetts, V. (1992). Fifteen-Month follow up with asthmatics utilizing EMG/Incentive inspirometer feedback. *Biofeedback and Self-Regulation, 17*(2), 143–151. https://doi.org/10.1007/BF01000104

[21]Fried, R. (1987). *The hyperventilation syndrome.* Baltimore: The Johns Hopkins University Press.

[22]Ley, R. (1991). The efficacy of breathing retraining and the centrality of hyperventilation in panic disorder: A reinterpretation of experimental findings. *Behavior Research & Therapy, 29*(3), 301–304. https://doi.org/10.1016/0005-7967(91)90121-I

[23]Castro, J. (2107). *Why do people "twitch" when falling asleep?* Retrieved December 30, 2018 from https://www.livescience.com/39225-why-people-twitch-falling-asleep.html

[24]Heide, F. J., & Borkovec, T. D. (1983). Relaxation-induced anxiety: Paradoxical anxiety enhancement due to relaxation training. *Journal of Consulting and Clinical Psychology, 51,* 171–182. https://doi.org/10.1037/0022-006X.51.2.171

[25]Newman M. G., LaFreniere, L. S., & Jacobson, N. C. (2018). Relaxation-induced anxiety: Effects of peak and trajectories of change on treatment outcome for generalized anxiety disorder. Psychotherapy Research, 4, 616–629. https://doi.org/10.1080/10503307.2016.1253891

[26]Bernstein, D. A., Borkovec, T. D., & Hazlett-Stevens, H. (2000). *New directions in progressive relaxation training. A guidebook for helping professionals.* Westport, CT: Praeger Publishers.

[27]Lundervold, D. A., Vick, L. B., Santoyo, J., Walsh, M., & Stern, E. R. (2010). *Acquisition and generalization of Behavioral Relaxation Training skills: Trainer and participant effects.* Association for Psychological Science. Boston, MA.

Supplement
Behavior Analyst Certification Board 5th Edition Task List

A. Philosophical Underpinnings
A-1 Identify the goals of behavior analysis as a science (i.e., description, prediction, control).
A-2 Explain the philosophical assumptions underlying the science of behavior analysis (e.g., selectionism, determinism, empiricism, parsimony, pragmatism).
A-3 Describe and explain behavior from the perspective of radical behaviorism.
A-4 Distinguish among behaviorism, the experimental analysis of behavior, applied behavior analysis, and professional practice guided by the science of behavior analysis.
A-5 Describe and define the dimensions of applied behavior analysis (Baer, Wolf, & Risley, (1968).

B. Concepts and Principles
B-1 Define and provide examples of behavior, response, and response class.
B-2 Define and provide examples of stimulus and stimulus class.
B-3 Define and provide examples of respondent and operant conditioning.
B-4 Define and provide examples of positive and negative reinforcement contingencies.
B-5 Define and provide examples of schedules of reinforcement.
B-10 Define and provide examples of stimulus control.

C. Measurement, Data Display, and Interpretation
C-1 Establish operational definitions of behavior.
C-2 Distinguish among direct, indirect, and product measures of behavior.
C-3 Measure occurrence (e.g., frequency, rate, percentage).
C-5 Measure form and strength of behavior (e.g., topography, magnitude).
C-6 Measure trials to criterion.
C-7 Design and implement sampling procedures (i.e., interval recording, time sampling).
C-8 Evaluate the validity and reliability of measurement procedures.

C-9 Select a measurement system to obtain representative data given the dimensions of behavior and the logistics of observing and recording.
C-10 Graph data to communicate relevant quantitative relations (e.g., equal-interval graphs, bar graphs, cumulative records).
C-11 Interpret graphed data.

D. Experimental Design
D-1 Distinguish between dependent and independent variables.
D-5 Use single-subject experimental designs (e.g., reversal, multiple baseline, multielement, changing criterion).

G. Behavior-Change Procedures
G-1 Use positive and negative reinforcement procedures to strengthen behavior.
G-5 Use modeling and imitation training.
G-6 Use instructions and rules.
G-9 Use discrete-trial, free-operant, and naturalistic teaching arrangements.
G-14 Use reinforcement procedures to weaken behavior (e.g., DRA, FCT, DRO, DRL, NCR).
G-17 Use token economies.
G-19 Use contingency contracting.

H. Selecting and Implementing Interventions
H-1 State intervention goals in observable and measurable terms.
H-4 When a target behavior is to be decreased, select an acceptable alternative behavior to be established or increased.
H-7 Make data-based decisions about the effectiveness of the intervention and the need for treatment revision.

I. Personnel Supervision and Management
I-4 Train personnel to competently perform assessment and intervention procedures.

Chapter 5
Neurodevelopmental Disorders

Neurodevelopmental disorders comprise a broad class of conditions, characterized by impairments in cognitive, emotional, perceptual, and motor behavior, that result from abnormal brain functioning. According to the American Psychiatric Association, neurologic-related deficits that have an onset between birth and eighteen years of age are termed *neurodevelopmental disorders*.[1] These include persons meeting diagnostic criteria for Intellectual Disability (ID), Autism Spectrum Disorder (ASD), Schizophrenic Spectrum Disorder (SSD), and Attention Deficit/Hyperactivity Disorder (ADHD).

The emphasis on normalization and deinstitutionalization has accomplished much in teaching self-care and vocational skills to persons with neurodevelopmental disorders. It is also apparent that such individuals could benefit from stress, anger, and anxiety management skills based on relaxation training.[2-9] For example, surveys indicate that persons with such disabilities suffer from a full range of emotional and behavioral problems and may actually be more susceptible to emotional disturbances than people without such disabilities.[10-17] For example, persons with schizophrenia are particularly vulnerable to stressful life events.[12] Also, the disruption and demands caused by relocation from an institution to a community living facility may be extremely stressful for people with such disabilities. These issues are more prevalent in recent years as the movement to community living and supported living arrangements has markedly increased.

Reform in placement options for persons with developmental disabilities and psychiatric issues was initiated in President Kennedy's 1964 mandate that established a network of federally-supported community mental health centers (CMHCs).[10] Funding for community-based services has waxed and waned since 1968. With the deinstitutionalization process finally taking root in the mid to late 1970's, individuals with disabilities began to reside in the community and were presented with a vast array of novel environments and expectations that were not present in the institution. Participating in schools, community living, and integrated employment with same age peers are significant stressors for individuals with disabilities. This chapter focuses on the application of BRT to manage stress, anxiety, anger, and other behavior problems in persons with neurodevelopment disabilities. We also describe how BRT procedures can be modified to be of the greatest benefit to the individual.

INTELLECTUAL DISABILITIES (ID)

Intellectual disability is characterized by deficits in mental functioning, often measured by intelligence tests, as well as a lack of or marked difficulty in learning everyday adaptive living skills. These limitations easily lead to problematic emotional behavior such as aggression or withdrawal.

BRT for Adults with ID

Bonnie McGimpsey[17] first demonstrated the feasibility of teaching relaxation to adults with ID using BRT procedures. Two men and two women (age range 21 to 44 years, Wechsler Adult Intelligence Scale (WAIS) IQ score range 67 to 79), who attended a sheltered workshop, were referred by their rehabilitation counselors. They were not diagnosed with particular stress or anxiety disorders, but their counselors judged that they could benefit from relaxation training. They were ambulatory and were not on psychotropic medication. Two of the participants were married to each other.

A multiple-baseline-across-behaviors design was employed in which training was introduced sequentially across the ten items of the BRS. This was replicated in each of the four participants. Baseline, post-training, and four-week follow-up sessions consisted of a ten-minute period during which participants were asked to sit quietly and relax but received no instruction or feedback, followed by a five-minute assessment period. Training occurred daily except weekends. Sessions were twenty-five to thirty minutes in duration, including five-minute adaptation, ten-minute training, and five-minute assessment periods. In addition to the BRS, frontalis and forearm flexor electromyographic (EMG) levels and self-report of relaxation measures, were obtained in each session.

During training, each new item was labeled and modeled, followed by a request that the participant imitate the relaxed behavior for fifteen to thirty seconds. Rehearsal trials, in which the participant demonstrated the current item, plus all previously trained behaviors, required a sixty-second criterion. When all ten items had been trained, proficiency training continued until the participant demonstrated 90 percent or better BRS scores for two consecutive sessions. No formal home practice or maintenance procedures were implemented because training took place every day. Reliability of BRS scoring was established with a trained observer behind a one-way window. Reliability ranged from 88 percent to 94 percent agreement between trainer and observer.

In general, behaviors unrelaxed prior to training showed rapid improvement with the onset of training. Breathing presented the most difficulty, perhaps in part because it was the last item trained and received the fewest trials. All ten behaviors were trained within four to six sessions, with an additional two to five sessions necessary to reach the proficiency criterion of 90%. There were some decrements in performance at the post-training and follow-up sessions, although not to baseline levels.

EMG levels were not consistently related to BRS scores. One participant showed a marked decrease in both frontalis and flexor EMG levels during BRT. A second participant showed frontal and flexor increases over baseline at the start of training, which declined as training progressed. A third participant showed a marked increase on the first day of proficiency training with a reduction to levels slightly below baseline thereafter. The fourth participant showed a marked increase in flexor tension at the beginning of training with a subsequent decline, whereas frontalis levels remained steady throughout training. Self-report measures for two participants were consistent with their BRS scores, with improved feelings of relaxation as training progressed. Self-report scores for a third participant fluctuated throughout training, both higher and lower than baseline. The fourth participant did not like the procedure and reported feeling quite tense by the end of training.

BRT for Children with ID

FEASIBILITY OF TEACHING RELAXATION TO CHILDREN WITH ID. Paclawski and Yoo[18] reported employing BRT with nineteen children with ID who were referred to the Neurobehavioral Unit of the Kennedy Kreiger Institute for evaluation for a variety of agitated or anxious behaviors. Prior to instruction, items that could serve as reinforcers were assessed, and a baseline session determined pre-training BRS scores and how long each child could sit quietly. Relaxed behaviors were taught by modeling, and a graduated prompt hierarchy of verbal, gestural, and physical guidance, as needed. Reinforcers were delivered contingent on correct imitation and maintenance. One to three behaviors were taught per session, depending on individual capabilities, to a mastery criterion of at least 80 percent over three consecutive sessions. Session duration was based on the baseline in-seat time. A random order of the ten target behaviors was employed for nine children, and a fixed order from large to small muscle groups was employed for the rest.

Overall, 89 percent (17 out of 19) of the children reached criterion. The fixed order of training was judged to be more effective—the two children who did not reach criterion were in the random group. The total time to reach criterion varied widely, from 12 to 520 minutes (M=124 minutes). The authors were encouraged to include BRT in their behavioral intervention programs and preliminary evidence suggested it enhanced outcomes in the treatment of maladaptive behavior in children with developmental disabilities.

BRT FOR A CHILD WITH ID AND HYPERVENTILATION-INDUCED SEIZURES. Keisel, Lutzker, and Campbell[19] employed a multiple-baseline-across-settings design to examine the functional relation between relaxation, hyperventilation, and seizure activity. Tim, a six-year-old child with profound intellectual disability, was able to name objects, mimic simple motor actions, and comply with simple commands. He had developed a seizure disorder at two years of age and began hyperventilating at age four after anti-seizure medication was started. Hyperventilation occurred when he became excited about an object or event, and often triggered a seizure. Observers were trained to reliably record hyperventilation and seizure behaviors in both home (for 30-minute periods) and school (60-minute periods) settings while Tim engaged in typical daily activities. No BRS measures of relaxation were obtained.

BRT was carried out in several rooms at home, using a recliner, sofa or bed. The list of ten relaxed behaviors was modified to focus on Tim's breathing; eyes were open and mouth closed, as hyperventilation occurred with an open mouth. Slow regular breathing through the nose was labeled "quiet mouth." Intervention was contingent on two hyperventilation breaths; Tim's mother would place him in the relaxed postures and instruct him, "Tim, listen, quiet mouth," at approximate five-second intervals. When hyperventilation ceased, he was praised and allowed to return to whatever activity he'd been engaged in. A second intervention occurred when Tim was ill with a virus and hyperventilation frequency increased. This consisted of five-to-ten-minute practice periods several times a day, in which his mother placed him in the BRT postures and provided consistent praise every five seconds for "quiet mouth." Spontaneous prompt fading occurred, in which his mother had only to say, "Tim...," and he would say, "quiet mouth," breathe through his nose, and place himself in the BRT positions. After hyperventilation and seizure episodes decreased and stabilized at home, intervention was implemented at school. Finally, monthly follow-up observations were conducted.

Table 5.1 shows the average number of occurrences of hyperventilation and seizure episodes during observation periods at home and school over the course of the study. The number of observations in each phase, and range of occurrences is given in in parentheses. Consistent with the multiple-baseline design, two baselines were conducted at school (labeled A and B); the first concurrent with baseline observations at home, and the second while intervention was implemented at home.

It is apparent that seizures did not follow every hyperventilation episode, occurring at roughly half to one-quarter the frequency. During baseline, hyperventilation and seizures occurred much more frequently at home compared to school, especially considering that the observation periods were twice as long at school. In fact, they occurred at very low rates during school baseline (A), but increased markedly during school baseline (B), when Intervention began at home. The authors do not address why decreasing these behaviors at home by use of contingent BRT might have a contrast effect of increasing them at school. Hyperventilation and seizures decreased at school with Intervention, and remained at low rates in both settings during follow-up. Social validation questionnaires were administered to Tim's

Table 5.1

Mean and range of hyperventilation and seizure episodes during observation periods at home and school for three phases of the study: Baseline, Intervention, and Follow-up; (n= the number of observation periods in each phase).

	HOME		
	Baseline (n=7)	*Intervention (n=12)*	*Follow-up (n=4)*
Mean Hypervent (Range)	13.14 (3–22)	5.50 (0–14)	2.25 (0–4)
Mean Seizure (Range)	7.14 (0–16)	0.75 (0–4)	0.0 (0–0)
	SCHOOL		
	Baseline (n=7)	*Intervention (n=12)*	*Follow-up (n=4)*
Mean Hypervent (Range)	A(*n*=8) B(*n*=5) 9.62 17.0 (2–17) (8–22)	8.60 (4–14)	5.50 (0–6)
Mean Seizure (Range)	1.75 5.40 (0–5) (4–8)	2.20 (0–6)	2.50 (2–3)

Based on Kiesel et al. (1989). Behavioral relaxation training to reduce hyperventilation and seizures in a profoundly retarded epileptic child. *Journal of the Multihandicapped Person*, 2(3) 179–190.

parents and teachers. All rated the intervention as highly acceptable and effective.

Anger and Aggression in Adults with ID

Surveys of persons with ID show that high rates of frustration, anger, and aggression occur across a variety of life circumstances.[14,15] The prevalence of aggression in the ID population has been shown to range from 10 to 23 percent for community samples and 37 to 40 percent for institutionalized samples.[16] Aggressive behavior takes a toll on the lives of family members living with persons with ID, often resulting in their placement in supervised living situations.[15] And the frequent aggressive behavior seen in residential and treatment settings has a negative impact on those caring for them.[18]

Lindsay and colleagues[20] incorporated BRT into a treatment program for mildly intellectually disabled (M WAIS IQ = 65.4 to 66.2) adults with severe anger and aggression. A between-groups research design, with a waiting-list control group, was used to determine the differences in anger management that could be achieved through the use of BRT. Thirty-three participants were trained in the intervention portion of the study. Forty sessions of anger-management training were conducted, in which BRT was part of the package. The first two sessions consisted of BRT followed by progressive muscle relaxation (PMR) and breathing-based relaxation. Three to four sessions were devoted to the relaxation and breathing retraining. Role play scenarios were used to provoke anger, during which the participants were taught to engage in the relaxation strategies to gain self-management skills. Generic and individualized anger-provoking scenarios were used. After the role-play, participants were asked to rate their level of anger on a Likert scale. Daily self-report anger ratings were also obtained. It is noteworthy that BRS scores indicating degree of relaxation skills were not reported.

Anger scores in the relaxation group declined from baseline to post-treatment. Daily self-report anger also showed significant decreases in the relaxation group compared to the control group. The study also found improvements in anger management for control subjects after they received the relaxation program.

Lindsay and colleagues[21] also reported a series of case studies that incorporated relaxation into the treatment programs of adults with ID and severe aggression. The case studies attempted to match the level of cognitive and behavioral challenge of the participant with the type and level of relaxation intervention. Three participants with WAIS IQ scores ranging from 40 to 69, took part. The relaxation strategy employed was individualized to best address the strengths of each participant. Only one of the three participants was trained using BRT.

Mr. G, a 42-year-old male, with a WAIS IQ score less than 40, displayed ritualistic behavior that culminated in extreme aggressive behavior if he was interrupted. Response prevention (extinction) procedures were employed to address his compulsive touching of objects. The emotional behavior he displayed as a result of the extinction procedure was addressed through the use of BRT. BRT was selected because initial assessments showed that learning the PMR procedure (i.e., tense-relax exercises and covert observation of muscle tension) was too challenging for him and might have led to increased aggression toward others. BRT was more appropriate because it was easier for him to focus on verbal instruction and differential reinforcement of overt behavior. Verbal and gestural prompts, modeling, and social reinforcement were used to teach the relaxed behaviors. The performance of the relaxed postures was paired with the phrase "be calm." To increase self-management skills, Mr. G was taught to engage in the relaxed behaviors when the verbal cue to relax was given.

A steady decline in the frequency of aggressive behavior occurred following BRT. Low levels of aggressive behavior were maintained six weeks and three months after the initiation of BRT. The verbal cue to relax allowed Mr. G to engage in increased self-management by using his relaxation skills.

Anxiety in Adults with ID

Lindsay and colleagues[21] also conducted a series of studies comparing BRT to other relaxation and control procedures in adults with ID and anxiety. Lindsay, Baty, Michie, and Richardson[22] examined the effect of four relaxation conditions. Fifty participants, evenly divided on sex, ranging in age from 25 to 69 years (M=43 years) with moderate to severe intellectual disabilities, participated. WAIS IQ scores ranged from 30 to 55 (M=44). All were judged to be extremely anxious and agitated, with restlessness, poor attention, and disruptive vocal and motor behaviors. Participants were randomly assigned to five groups, with five men and five women in each.

There were four relaxation conditions: two employing BRT (one group and one individual training); and two employing PMR (onr group and one individual training); as well as a no-treatment control group. Daily individual training sessions, 30 to 45 minutes in duration, were conducted five days a week for a total of twelve training sessions. Group sessions were twice as long as individual training. Assessments were carried out by raters blind to treatment conditions in sessions over three-day periods prior to training, midway through training, and at the completion of training. A modified nine-item (breathing was excluded) BRS ratings scale was used to assess relaxed behavior. Instead of a binary present or absent score, the nine behaviors were rated on a five-point scale with anchors of *completely relaxed* to *very anxious*; a tenth item, "general relaxation/tension," was included. The item ratings were summed to obtain a score on a "behavioral anxiety scale." Inter-rater agreement on this measure, within one scale point, was about 88 percent. Pulse rates also were measured at the time of the behavioral rating.

A two-way analysis of variance with repeated measures of the "anxiety" score indicated significant main effects of training, group assignment, and a significant training x assignment interaction. All relaxation groups showed improvements over the course of training, with the no-treatment group showing no change. The individual BRT group had the greatest improvement, differing significantly from both PMR groups, and showed near maximal effects after only six training sessions. Group BRT training was midway between individual BRT and individual PMR training groups. Group BRT was not statistically different from individual BRT or PMR. Group BRT was better than group PMR. No significant main effect for pulse rate was observed, although a significant interaction was found, showing a significant decrease in heart rate for the individual BRT group.

Lindsay et al.[22] concluded that group BRT was a cost-effective way of teaching relaxation to persons with moderate to severe intellectual disabilities. They found BRT effects were achieved more rapidly than with PMR, and that the participants had particular difficulty with PMR in a group setting. This study did not measure the influence of relaxation on other areas of the participants' lives, but subsequent investigations examined the effects of BRT on various performance measures.

Anxiety and Cognitive Deficits in Adults with ID

Lindsay and Morrison[24] measured the performance of persons with ID on cognitive tasks that were thought to be influenced negatively by anxious arousal. A total of twenty adult participants (age and gender not specified) with WAIS IQ scores below 55 were selected because of problems related to agitation and anxiety such as pacing, vocal outbursts, and stereotyped mannerisms and verbalizations.

Participants were randomly assigned to two groups of ten persons each. Individuals in one group were given twelve sessions of BRT, whereas those in the control group sat in comfortable chairs for comparable periods and were read stories from a children's book. Immediately after each relaxation or story session, participants were tested on digit span, incidental learning, and general knowledge. The digit span test assesses immediate recall and attention capacity. Increasingly longer strings of random numbers were vocally presented, commencing with one digit, then two digits, and so on. Any correct repetition was scored positively. The incidental learning task required participants to insert up to ten colored pegs on a pegboard, changing direction (right, left, up, or down) after every third peg; participants were then asked to recall the colors of the last three pegs. The general knowledge test was based on a pool of thirty questions concerning common objects and daily routines. Mean performance scores on each measure were compared from Pre-Training (three baseline sessions), Mid-Training (session five to seven), and Late-Training (session ten to twelve), for the two groups.

Statistical analysis (two-way analysis of variance with repeated measures over time) showed that the BRT group steadily improved from Pre, to Mid, to Late-Training on both the digit span and incidental learning tasks, whereas the control group showed no changes. On the general knowledge test, both groups were comparable, with no change over time.

Performance on digit span and incidental learning was hypothesized to be related to working memory, which was impaired by increased arousal and anxiety, and hence was improved by relaxation. General knowledge was related to long-term storage and was not affected by anxiety or relaxation. Thus, laboratory measures of cognitive functioning were enhanced by BRT in persons with intellectual disability and anxiety.

The authors recognized that no independent measure of anxiety was included; indeed, much of their speculation concerned internal states and processes. In more behavioral terms, BRT, which focuses on motor behavior, was found to have beneficial effects on observational and verbal behavior. Unfortunately, no measurement of relaxation was included in this study. Previous research[18] showed that BRT produced improvements on a behavioral anxiety scale, derived from the BRS, and one assumes that similar improvements occurred in the present study. Finally, the authors provided anecdotal evidence that persons trained in BRT were reported by ward staff to be less distractible and more engaged in other learning situations in their daily environments. These promising observations await more systematic investigation and suggest that BRT may be of value to individuals with subjective complaints of anxiety and memory problems.

Anxiety and Occupational Therapy Tasks in Adults with ID

The effect of BRT on performance during occupational therapy was examined to provide an indication of the usefulness of relaxation in the daily lives of persons with ID.[27] Three men and two women participants, ranging in age from 29 to 48 years, with WAIS IQ < 40, displayed a variety of agitated and anxious behaviors, such as shouting, inappropriate vocalizations, pacing, restlessness, and various facial and bodily mannerisms. These tended to increase in frequency when they were approached by other persons.

A clinical series approach to evaluation and treatment employing a multi-phase design over total of thirty sessions was conducted. All participants began with five baseline sessions in which they were simply asked to sit and relax. Two participants then received BRT for five sessions; on the sixth session, the cue words "quiet" and "still" were vocally introduced and paired with the relaxed behaviors. Over the next eight sessions, the amount of BRT instruction and feedback was progressively reduced. The final phase was "cue only," in which the participants were given only the vocal cue and no BRT instruction. The other three participants began with a cue-only phase for five sessions. They then received a BRT instruction phase, BRT paired with the cue words, and a final cue-only phase. After each session, participants were provided with twenty minutes of simple occupational therapy tasks, requiring color or shape matching and object manipulation. In addition, a new therapist was introduced at various times to determine whether relaxation effects were specific to the presence of the particular trainer or would be disrupted by the presence of a new person.

Participants were videotaped at the conclusion of each relaxation period and during occupational therapy. Independent raters scored the tapes according to the behavioral anxiety scale described earlier.[20] Raters also measured the amount of time "on-task," defined as "meaningful manipulation of the occupational materials." High levels of inter-observer agreement were reported for both measures.

Anxiety ratings declined markedly only when BRT was introduced; there were no changes during baseline or when cue words were introduced prior to BRT. Anxiety ratings remained low or continued to decrease when the cue words were paired with BRT and remained at low levels for all participants during the final cue-only phase. Introduction of a new therapist, or the return on a previous one had no disruptive effect on anxiety ratings. The amount of time spent on-task generally mirrored the anxiety ratings, remaining low during baseline and cue-only phases, increasing during the BRT and BRT-plus-cue-word phases, and staying at high levels during the final cue-only phase.

The authors concluded that the cue words by themselves had little effect in regulating the participant's behavior, but could be discriminative for relaxation after pairing with BRT and differential reinforcement procedures. Certainly, relaxed behaviors were maintained when BRT instruction was faded, but the role of the cue words in maintaining relaxation was not clearly demonstrated. This would require comparison to participants for whom BRT instruction was faded but no cue words were supplied. Individuals with normal intellectual functioning routinely maintain relaxed behavior in the absence of explicit cue words, although the role of covert self-instructions cannot be ruled out. It is likely that people with intellectual deficits may need external verbal prompts, or explicit training in self-instructions, to maintain a skill or use it in a new situation. For example, self-instructions were found to increase on-task behavior in two children with ID.[28] Lindsay et al.[27] did not mention whether they observed the participants using the cue words during relaxation practice or occupational therapy.

Teaching the verbal component of relaxation would seem to be an important factor in the maintenance and transfer of relaxed behaviors in other modalities. Lundervold[29] described teaching a woman with mild intellectual disability to repeat the ten labels of the relaxed behaviors to herself as a form of self-instruction, suggesting that this aided her in learning relaxation. Further research on relaxation and self-instruction with the ID population is warranted.

Summary

Studies have shown that persons with ID can learn relaxation skills by a variety of training methods.[3,5,7] Research by Lindsay and colleagues[20-27] indicate that BRT is relatively easy for such persons to learn, and that BRT can be taught in a group format, a very efficient approach for facilities with staff limitations. BRT has been shown to improve performance on short-term memory tests and on-task behavior. The results of several case studies suggest that BRT has positive effects on agitated, disruptive, and/or aggressive behavior among individuals with ID, though more controlled research is needed. Keisel et al.[19] demonstrated that BRT was effective in managing a chronic seizure disorder induced by the hyperventilation of a young child with significant ID. Because seizures are prevalent in individuals with ID, application of BRT in the chain of precursor behaviors appears useful. Much more work in this area is needed.

AUTISM SPECTRUM DISORDER (ASD)

Considerable evidence indicates that anxiety is a prevalent comorbid disorder related to autism spectrum disorder (ASD). Current estimates of the prevalence of comorbid anxiety disorders among individuals with ASD range between 42 percent and 55 percent.[30-32] To place this into perspective, the prevalence of anxiety disorders in typically developing children is in the 2 percent to 27 percent range.[33] Anxiety disorders among individuals with ASD are twice the rate seen in children without an ASD.[33] Social anxiety disorder represents a large portion of this group, with estimates near 29 percent.[31] In adults with ASD, the prevalence of co-occurring psychiatric disorders is close to 70 percent.[34] As with anyone, anxiety can pose a significant obstacle to social, vocational, and academic success. For people with ASD, anxiety also negatively impacts the extent to which they can be fully integrated into society. Despite such findings, treatment of persons with ASD and various related disabilities has received relatively little professional attention.[35-38]

Behavior Therapy for Anxiety in Children with ASD

Relaxation training has been one aspect of multi-component treatment in cognitive behavior therapy treatment packages for children diagnosed with High Functioning ASD and various anxiety disorders.[35-38] Relaxation training has been one aspect of multi-component cognitive behavior therapy treatment packages for children diagnosed with High Functioning ASD and various anxiety disorders. The treatment packages include training to recognize anxiety situations and reactions, cognitive restructuring, coping self-talk, exposure to feared stimuli, relaxation training, and a token economy. Procedures were also modified to accommodate the learning styles and limitations of children with ASD.

Results are very promising, but they do not show the extent to which the children learned relaxation or its contribution to the outcome.[38]

Young Adults with Anxiety and ASD

Bechtler[39] reported using BRT with two female college students, age 19 and 29, having ASD and comorbid anxiety. The BRS was used as a measure of overt relaxed behavior, and heart rate (HR) was assessed as a visceral response related to anxiety. The participants received four twice-weekly sessions of BRT, each lasting approximately thirty minutes, using the standard training format. All ten relaxed behaviors were taught in the first session. Seven sessions of proficiency training were then conducted. Mean interobserver agreement on relaxed behavior ranged from 95 to 98 percent.

Both participants acquired the relaxed behaviors very quickly. Participant 1 displayed a mean BRS score of 59 percent during baseline, improving to 85 percent after training. For Participant 2, BRS scores improved from 26 percent in baseline to 84 percent. Heart rate decreased following BRT for both participants. Mean baseline HR for Participant 1 was 95 bpm, which declined to 87 bpm following BRT. A similar result was observed for Participant 2, with HR decreasing from 80 bpm in baseline to 77 after BRT.

Participants were asked to rate their tension following home practice on a daily basis. Participant 2 reported a decrease in tension but Participant 1 did not comply with the request to practice or record. This study demonstrated that young adults with ASD can learn relaxation with BRT fairly easily, but little effort was made to apply those skills in situations evoking anxiety reactions.

Summary

Only very preliminary results are available to show the effectiveness of relaxation for persons with ASD and comorbid disorders. Chalfant et al. and other investigators[35-38] indicate that a comprehensive anxiety-management program is very helpful for children with HF-ASD, but the amount that relaxation contributed to that outcome is not clear. Bechtler[39] showed that adults can learn to relax via BRT very easily. However participants must be taught how to implement their relaxation skills in stressful situations for it to have a positive impact on their lives.

SCHIZOPHRENIC SPECTRUM DISORDER (SSD)

Current views of schizophrenia regard it as a disease characterized by cognitive, psychophysiological, and interpersonal deficits that result in a marked vulnerability to stress.[40-43] A number of studies indicate that psychotic episodes are more likely during periods of stressful life events and that persons experiencing them characterized by high levels of arousal.[42, 44] Accordingly, various relaxation training methods have been tried with persons diagnosed with schizophrenia including PMR, EMG biofeedback, and meditation.[45-49] Reduced EMG levels and improvements on self-reported anxiety and clinical rating measures have been reported. Although promising, there is little to recommend one method over another and there is no evidence of the use of relaxation *in vivo* to manage stress and anxiety or prevent relapse. For the reasons of simplicity and ease of training described previously, the use of BRT has been explored with this population.

Anxiety in Adults with SSD

Noe[50] investigated the effects of BRT with nine men in an independent community living program. They were recommended by their treatment coordinators as having high levels of anxiety, and each man volunteered to participate when the program was explained to him. They ranged in age from 23 to 54 years, and met *Diagnostic and Statistical Manual* criteria for chronic schizophrenia. They were part of a university-affiliated independent living skills program in a large urban area. Most had histories of other problems including substance abuse, obsessive-compulsive disorder, extrapyramidal symptoms, tardive dyskinesia, intellectual disabilities, or criminal activity. All were taking psychotropic medications.

A multiple-probe-across-participants design was employed, with three cohorts of three men in each. During baseline, participants were asked to relax in a reclining chair in their usual fashion for about fifteen minutes. Acquisition training was conducted daily to a criterion of a BRS score of at least 80 percent relaxed for two successive sessions, with a minimum of four sessions. On reaching the criterion, the men were placed in a maintenance phase in which they had weekly assessment sessions; if they fell below 80 percent relaxed during maintenance, they received immediate "booster" training. Follow-up assessments were conducted two, four, and six weeks after the conclusion of maintenance. All sessions were videotaped.

Participants were instructed to practice BRT at home at least ten minutes daily; each was given a large sign with the word "RELAX" to post in his apartment and a home practice sheet to fill out and return to the investigator. The men received various reinforcing consequences for participating. For completing a session each man received a soda and candy bar; for completing acquisition, he received a cassette tape or tape player; for two consecutive maintenance and follow-up sessions at 80 percent or better, he received a T-shirt, hat, or sweatpants of his choice; and at the completion of the study, each man received $10 and dinner at a restaurant with the researcher.

The BRS was scored for a five-minute period at the conclusion of each session. Bilateral trapezius EMG and electrodermal (EDR) activity in the right hand was measured concurrently. (The trapezius was chosen based on pilot research that indicated this site to be the most active.) The State Anxiety Inventory,[51] a structured self-report instrument, and the Brief Psychiatric Rating Scale (BPRS),[52] a structured clinical interview, were completed at two-week intervals. Reliability of BRS scoring was determined by a trained independent observer, blind to the study phase, who scored 25 percent of the videotaped observation periods; agreement ranged from 80 percent to 96 percent and averaged 87 percent. Reliability of BPRS scoring was determined in a similar fashion; agreement ranged from 75 percent to 92 percent and averaged 85 percent.

The findings were fairly similar across individuals. Their data are aggregated in Table 5.2, which shows the means and ranges of scores on the dependent measures in baseline, acquisition, maintenance, and follow-up phases. Five participants reached the BRS acquisition criterion of 80 percent or better in the minimum four sessions, and no one required more than seven.

BRS scores were maintained at 80 percent or better for eight of nine men. EMG levels were fairly low during baseline and did not change during train-

Table 5.2
Mean scores on measures across experimental conditions.

	Condition			
Measure	*Baseline*	*Acquisition*	*Maintenance*	*Follow-up*
Behavioral Relaxation Scale (BRS)	26	78	80	82
EMG in Microvolts (mV)	1.1mV	1.2mV	1.3mV	1.1mV
State Anxiety Inventory	43.6	35.1	35.8	34.4
Brief Psychiatric Ratings Scale	44.4	38.4	35.7	33.5

Based on Noe, S. R. (1997). Behavioral relaxation training to reduce autonomic hyperarousal in individuals with schizophrenia. Unpublished doctoral dissertation, Southern Illinois University at Carbondale.

ing. Similarly, EDR levels were generally low and consistent from baseline to training phases. Anxiety scores decreased from baseline levels for all participants; five of nine participants scored about the mean for a psychiatric population during baseline, whereas only one person did so by follow-up. BPRS scores showed similar improvements, with all participants having a decrease in ratings of their psychiatric symptoms. Five participants consistently returned their home practice sheets and four did not; there was no difference in any of the measures of those who reported practicing.

This study demonstrated that outpatients with chronic schizophrenia could easily learn and maintain relaxed behavior and that this was associated with decreases in self-reported anxiety and other symptoms. Adjustments were made in BRS—including diaphragmatic breathing, progressive temporal requirements, and postural definitions—to meet the needs of individual participants. In contrast to other studies with this population, attrition did not occur. A major factor may have been the rich schedule of tangible and social reinforcers for participating and meeting goals. The reinforcers also may have contributed to the decrease in reported symptoms apart from any relaxation effect. Further research on this issue is needed.

Bizarre ideation sometimes intruded; for example, one man did not want to open his mouth for fear that a cockroach would crawl in. Consistent with other research,[47] hallucinations and obsessive thoughts did not appear to interfere with relaxation, nor did they decrease. BRT did not provide strong enough verbal and observational behavior alternatives to overcome these problems.

The low baseline levels on physiological measures may have created a "floor effect" that prevented improvement. Reasons for these low initial levels remain speculative. The long-term goal of relaxation training in this population is to provide them with a means of coping with stressful events that could trigger a relapse. Preliminary data suggested some decrement in relapse rates; only one person had a "crisis" requiring interventions after BRT, but longer term follow-up is needed. To be truly effective, participants would need to be taught to use relaxation and other coping responses when they begin to become upset. Research on such a program is warranted.

Summary

While Noe demonstrated that men diagnosed with schizophrenia can learn relaxation via BRT and a rich reinforcement schedule and that this is associated with reductions in scores on anxiety scales, it is only a beginning. It remains to be seen if they can learn to engage in relaxation skills during stressful situations that evoke anxiety and aggression. As in programs with individuals with ID, transfer of relaxed behaviors to upsetting environments would need to be specifically taught. Also unknown is the extent to which symptoms such as hallucinations interfere with relaxed behavior, or, perhaps, vice versa.

ATTENTION-DEFICIT/HYPERACTIVITY DISORDER (ADHD)

Attention-deficit/hyperactivity disorder (ADHD) is a prevalent neurodevelopmental disorder, with estimates of one in 20 children and adolescents in the United States meeting diagnostic criteria.[53] Prevalence rates have increased from 6.1 percent to 10.2 percent from 1997 to 2016.[54] Nearly 80 percent of children with ADHD continue to meet criteria as adolescents, with growing evidence of ADHD-related behavior continuing into adulthood.[54] People with ADHD tend to have lower occupational status, poor social relationships, and are more likely to commit driving offenses and develop substance abuse.[55,56] Parents and siblings also suffer as a result of the behavioral problems associated with ADHD; increased levels of stress in family members are common, as are depression and marital discord.[57-59]

Children with hyperactivity are characterized as impulsive, overactive, incapable of sustained attention, socially disruptive, and poor students. Stimulant medication, which has a "paradoxical" calming effect in many children, is by far the most common treatment. Side effects of stimulant medication include decreased appetite, cardiovascular problems, insomnia, irritability, weight loss, headache, and upper abdominal pain.[60-62] Side effects of stimulant medication appear to be worse for children with ID and ADHD.[60]

Long-term drug use has raised serious objections because of growth retardation and lack of academic progress in medicated children.[60]

BRT for Children with ADHD

Relaxation training may be a benign substitute for medication. Raymer and Poppen[63] reviewed several studies that reported positive effects of frontalis EMG biofeedback or PMR on measures such as parent rating scales, psychological tests, and academic and psychomotor tasks. Other research found such training methods to be no more effective than attention control in improving performance.

Rick Raymer adapted BRT for use with three children having ADHD, showing its feasibility for use with this population, and demonstrated some benefits that may result. Participant 1, 11 years old, lived in a group home because of family problems with his behavior; he was taking ten milligrams of Ritalin daily at the start of the study. Participant 2, nine years old, was referred by his physician; Ritalin had not improved his behavior, and his parents were reluctant to reinstate drug treatment. Participant 3, nine years old, was referred by his school because of poor performance; he had a history of taking Ritalin, but his parents objected to his continuing its use. All boys met the diagnostic criteria of Barkley[64] and had been diagnosed as hyperactive by at least one physician.

EMG monitoring equipment was first demonstrated to the boys and then kept out of sight. Reliability observations, for at least 25 percent of the sessions with each child, were made through a one-way window by a trained observer in an adjacent room. Agreement between observer and trainer was better than 90 percent for each child.

Training sessions were conducted approximately twice a week. A multiple-probe-across-participants design was employed. Measures included the BRS, frontalis EMG levels, parent ratings on the Hyperactivity Index of the Conners Questionnaire,[65] and self-report in which the boys were asked, "Answer yes or no: Do you feel relaxed?" BRT was modified by awarding tokens (poker chips) for approximations. to relaxed behaviors, such as lying in the recliner and listening to the trainer. Later they were contingent on performance of relaxed behaviors for specified periods of time. The tokens were dropped into a can where they made an audible clink, and did not interfere with relaxation. Tokens were spent after each session on an outing or treat provided by the trainer.

After reaching the acquisition criterion, Participant 1 had difficulty meeting the proficiency criterion. During an outing, the trainer noticed that the child sat quietly in a beanbag chair. Reasoning that the beanbag provided better body support than the big recliner, a beanbag was employed in the next session with an immediate improvement in relaxed behaviors. After the child reach proficiency criterion, a reversal to the recliner was conducted and then back to the beanbag. The same procedure was followed for Participants 2 and 3.

Follow-up measurements were conducted two to three months after training, at which time the parents were offered the opportunity to learn the procedure in their homes. All parents agreed to the program, including purchasing beanbag chairs and implementing token reinforcement. For each participant, the trainer first conducted an initial home baseline session. Next, the mother was trained briefly in this relaxed behavior herself and observed the trainer conduct BRT and BRS scoring with her child. During the third and fourth sessions, the mother conducted BRT, following prompts provided by the trainer. Thereafter, the mother conducted BRT for ten consecutive days with the trainer observing on the first, fifth, and tenth days. A final follow-up measurement session was conducted in the home a month later.

BRS scores for all three boys are shown in Figure 5.1. They displayed low variable rates of relaxed behaviors at baseline with no improvement. Scores increased with the onset of BRT, but plateaus were reached between 40 percent and 70 percent relaxed. Introduction of the beanbag chair resulted in rapid achievement of the proficiency criterion (80 percent or better for two consecutive sessions) for all boys. A reversal session in the recliner disrupted BRS scores, but they rapidly recovered when the beanbag was reinstated.

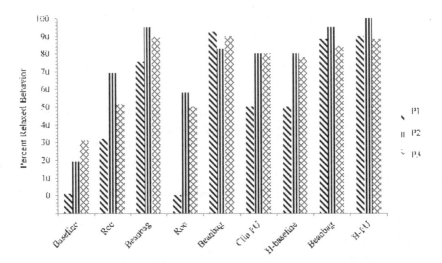

Figure 5.1 Behavioral Relaxation Scale (BRS) scores for three boys with hyperactivity disorder.
Based on Raymer, H. R. & Poppen, R. (1985) Behavioral relaxation training with hyperactive children, *Journal of Behavior Therapy and Experimental Psychiatry*, 16, 309–316.

Some decrement at one-month follow-up was noted, particularly for Participant 1, who was given a booster session in which he was instructed to "relax like you were taught," resulting in immediate improvement.

Decreases in BRS scores occurred for all three boys in the initial home baseline sessions. Performance improved immediately with training by the mothers and was maintained at the last follow-up. Frontalis EMG data for each child showed a strong relationship to the BRS scores, declining as BRS improved (see Figure 5.2). For Participant 3, EMG levels improved only slightly until the beanbag was implemented. Reversal effects are obvious for all three boys. EMG levels increased markedly during the home baseline sessions but declined rapidly when mothers implemented BRT and were maintained at low levels at follow-up. Correlations between BRS scores and EMG levels were -42 ($p < .05$) for Participant 1, $-.56$ ($p < .05$) for Participant 2, and $-.81$ ($p < .001$) for Participant 3.

Parent ratings on the Hyperactivity Index of the Conners Questionnaire indicated the ratings at the first follow-up were about one standard deviation lower than those at the end of baseline; however, these scores still were within the "hyperactive" range. Scores for all three children improved markedly immediately after home training by the mothers. All were within the "normal" range at the final home follow-up. In addition to these formal mea-

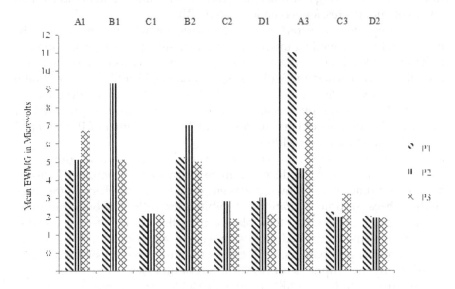

Figure 5.2 Mean EMG across phases for three boys with hyperactivity disorder.
Based on Raymer, H. R. & Poppen, R. (1985) Behavioral relaxation training with hyperactive children, *Journal of Behavior Therapy and Experimental Psychiatry, 16*, 309–316.

sures, the parents were asked about their reactions to the procedures. All reported that it was convenient and easily implemented and that they felt it had benefited their children. They reported things such as a child employing the procedures on his own while watching television or showing off his skills for relatives. All children reported that they felt relaxed on every session, including baseline. This was taken as an indication that their verbal reports were related to the social contingencies rather than to their feelings of relaxation.

Although no formal efforts were made to transfer the skills to the home environment during the office training phase, some improvements on the Hyperactivity Index were reported by all parents. When home practice was implemented, marked improvements on this measure were noted. This may reflect actual changes in children's comportment at home due to relaxation, or it may have altered the parents' perception of their children. Objective observation of child behavior in the home would need to address this question.

Teaching Parents to Teach BRT

Donney[66] systematically replicated Raymer's findings by teaching parents to conduct BRT in their own homes right from the beginning. This avoided the problem of transferring training to the home environment and demonstrated how easily nonprofessionals can learn to do BRT.

Three boys were referred by their pediatricians who judged them to be inadequately controlled by medication. Participant 1 (8 years) was taking 25 milligrams of Ritalin daily. Participant 2 (10 years), was taking 20 milligrams of Ritalin daily. Participant 3, (9 years), was taking 15 milligrams of Ritalin daily. In addition to medical diagnosis, the boys met the criteria described in Barkley.[64] Two families purchased beanbag chairs, and one was provided for the third. The mothers of Participants 1 and 2 and the father of Participant 3 engaged in training their children.

Training and observation were conducted in each child's room or the family room with efforts made to minimize distractions. A simple A-B design (baseline-training) with follow-up was employed, replicated across the three children, because time limitations prohibited the more elaborate multiple-baseline approach. Training took place during the summer school vacation months. Sessions were scheduled twice weekly, depending on the commitments of trainer and parents. Each child's training program suffered one or more lengthy interruptions due to vacations or illnesses.

Measures included the BRS, frontalis EMG levels, and parent ratings on the Hyperactivity Index of the Conners Questionnaire.[65] Prior to training and at follow-up, the Home Situations Questionnaire was filled out by the parents and the School Situations Questionnaire was filled out by the boys' schoolteachers. Classroom observations were conducted for Participant 2 on three behaviors ("out of seat," "talking out," and "on-task") by a teacher's assistant during baseline and by the trainer after treatment because the assistant no longer was available. On 25 percent of the sessions, another trained observer accompanied the trainer to measure reliability of the BRS.

For each participant, four baseline sessions were conducted with the trainer and parent both present. The child was asked to sit quietly for 20 minutes; the last five minutes comprised the measurement period for scoring the BRS and recording EMG levels. After each baseline session, the trainer and parent discussed the BRS scoring. The parent was given a copy of the BRS definitions and practiced the relaxed behaviors him or herself while the trainer provided feedback, guidance, and praise. Next, the trainer modeled relaxed and unrelaxed behaviors while the parent provided feedback.

Training sessions consisted of five minutes of adaptation, twenty minutes of BRT, and five minutes of assessment. The first three behaviors were taught by the trainer, while the parent observed and scored during the assessment period. Training was conducted similar to Raymer's procedure, including delivery of tokens for successful behavior. The trainer and parent reviewed their BRS Score Sheets after each session, and corrective feedback was given for discrepancies. The next two behaviors were taught by the parent, guided by silent signals from the trainer. The trainer kept track of the observation schedule and indicated to the parent which behaviors were unrelaxed by pointing to her own body. The last five behaviors were taught by the parent alone with the trainer providing corrective feedback after the session if needed.

After all ten items has been completed, proficiency training was conducted by the parent to a criterion of two successive sessions of 80 percent relaxed behaviors during the assessment period. The trainer's role at this point was to conduct BRS and EMG assessments and to provide feedback and encouragement. Tokens were spent by the child as soon after the session as possible on small treats and outings delivered by the parents. Throughout training, the families were encouraged to practice on their own, although no systematic data were collected. Two follow-up assessment sessions were conducted at one and three months.

Figure 5.3 shows the BRS scores for these children. There was no improvement during baseline; if anything, performance worsened. When BRT was implemented, the boys learned the 10 items within five to seven sessions. Participant 3 reached the proficiency criterion in four additional sessions, whereas Participant 1 required 12 more sessions. Agreement on BRS scores ranged between 90 and 93 percent for trainer and observer and between 87 and 95 percent for trainer and parents, indicating that the parents became proficient scorers of the BRS.

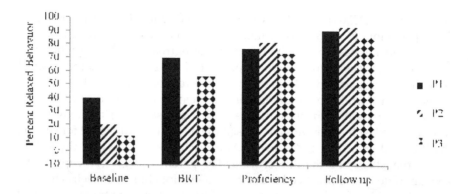

Figure 5.3. Mean BRS score for three boys with hyperactivity disorder trained by their parents.
Based on V. K. Donney & Poppen, R. (1989). Teaching parents to conduct behavioral relaxation training with their hyperactive children, *Journal of Behavior Therapy and Experimental Psychiatry, 20,* 319–325.

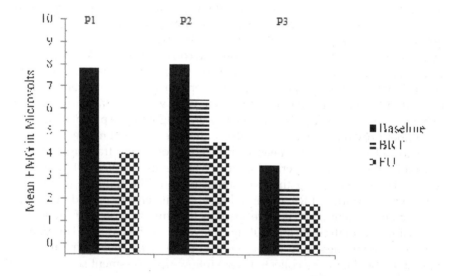

Figure 5.4. Mean frontalis EMG levels for three boys with hyperactivity across experimental conditions.
Based on V. K. Donney & Poppen, R. (1989). Teaching parents to conduct behavioral relaxation training with their hyperactive children, *Journal of Behavior Therapy and Experimental Psychiatry, 20,* 319–325.

Mean frontalis EMG levels during the assessment periods are shown in Figure 5.4. Baseline values were generally high and variable for Participants 1 and 2 but showed a systematic decline for Participant 3. During BRT, EMG values declined for all children and remained at low levels at follow-up. As in the previous study, EMG levels generally paralleled the BRS scores, decreasing as relaxed behavior increased. Correlations between these two measures were $-.72$ ($p < .001$) for Participant 1 and $-.61$ ($p < .01$) for Participant 3. The correlation for Participant 2 was not significant because of the unaccountably high EMG values in the fifteenth and seventeenth sessions.

Each child evidenced an improvement (decreased score) on the Conners scale in the follow-up as compared to the baseline period based. However, changes during the BRT period differed. The scores for Participant 1 actually increased slightly during BRT, indicating worsening behavior, but at follow-up his scores declined to within the "normal" range. Participant 2 showed no change during training and a small improvement by the follow-up period, remaining in the "hyperactive" range. Participant 3 had ratings in the "normal" range during baseline and showed an improvement during BRT that was maintained at follow-up.

For each child, the parents reported a marked improvement by follow-up, both in the percentage of situations reported as presenting a problem and in the severity rating of those situations. The same was not observed in the School Situations Questionnaire. It should be pointed out that the teachers doing the post–training ratings were different from the ones doing the initial rating because the children had gone to a higher grade, and so there are many confounding variables in these ratings. Participant 1 was rated as increasing in percentage of problem situations, although the severity rating decreased. Participant 3 was rated as improving in both percentage of situations and severity. Participant 2 was rated as increasing in both percentage and severity. This child's teacher, on learning of his diagnosis, tried to have him moved to a special classroom, even though classroom observations indicated that the percentage of intervals he was observed to be "talking out" decreased from 23 percent to 8 percent, "out of seat" decreased from 20 percent to one percent, and "on-task" increased from 23 percent to 86 percent.

This study demonstrated that parents quickly and easily learned to conduct BRT with their hyperactive children, essentially conducting training on their own after the third session. The objective criteria for relaxed behavior allowed the parents to easily observe their children and reinforce their children's performance. The parents reported that they did not maintain a formal training program; however, the children maintained the relaxed behaviors at least two months after training, and the parents gave anecdotal reports that they spontaneously engaged in relaxation.

Summary

Some comparisons between the Donney and Raymer study are in order. First, there were no differences in the number of sessions required to reach a proficiency criterion on the BRS. It was thought that using a beanbag chair from the outset would speed up acquisition. Perhaps this advantage was offset by the fact that parents were conducting training, but it was more likely that reaching the criterion was delayed by interruptions that occurred in the training regime as the children took time off to visit their grandmother or a divorced parent or to recover from an illness or injury.

Second, it was felt that conducting training in the home would facilitate general improvements in comportment, as measured by ratings on the Conners Questionnaire.[65] Improvements on the Hyperactivity Index during training occurred only for Participant 3, who was not very disruptive from the start. Improvements were noted for the other two children, but only at follow-up. The lack of improvement during the training phase may reflect the fact that the children were home all day every day; improved parental ratings occurred only at follow-up after the children were back in school.

A third point is that none of the parents maintained training after the formal program was over, although all felt that it had done much good for their children. These results point up the importance of training for maintenance, perhaps through a fading and follow-up program.

EMOTIONAL DISTURBANCE (ED)

Children and adolescents with serious emotional disturbance (ED) are members of a heterogeneous group with chronic functional impairments across settings. Adolescents labeled as "externalizing" demonstrate behavioral excesses such as anger, aggression, impulsiveness, property destruction and rule violation.[67] They are at high risk of having difficulties at home and school, developing substance abuse disorders and becoming involved in the juvenile justice system.[68,69]

Social Skills and Relaxation Training for Adolescents with ED

Baum and colleagues[70] reviewed the literature showing that socially deviant behavior is related to social skill deficits, and that heightened physiological arousal may potentiate aggressive and other impulsive behavior. Accordingly, they implemented a treatment package that included role-play, self-instruction, and relaxation (BRT augmented by PMR, imagery, and a cue word) with four males (ages 12 to 14) enrolled in a day treatment program. Monetary rewards were given for participation and achievement of certain goals. They employed a multiple-baseline-across-participants research design.

Relaxation was assessed via BRS, frontalis EMG, and pulse rate plethysmograph. Social skills were measured by observation of training videotapes of four operationally-defined behaviors (out of the twelve taught). Disruptive classroom behavior was measured by time-sampling direct observation of three target behaviors. Inter-observer reliability for all dependent measures was very high. The Conners Teacher Rating Scale[65] was completed pre- and post-treatment, with teachers blind to treatment conditions.

Results showed that BRS scores markedly improved with training for all participants, and that EMG and pulse-rate measures declined accordingly for three of the four boys. Social-skill scores improved during training and generalized to a novel role-play scenario for everyone. There were no consistent changes in frequency of classroom disruptive behavior, but the authors suggest that perhaps the time-sampling procedure was not sensitive enough. On the other hand, marked increases in the trained social skills were observed in the classroom for three of the students. Teacher ratings on the Conners showed some improvements on some of the sub-scales.

Summary

Consistent with reports described for other populations, relaxed behaviors were easily acquired by the students with ED. BRT was taught first due to the ease of learning, and PMR appears to have been added to give a "boost" to the treatment effect of BRT, though the work of Schilling and Poppen[71] suggests that little is to be gained relative to BRT by itself. Further work in this area is needed.

The treatment package was effective in teaching social skills, though the precise contribution of PMR or BRT is unclear. Relaxation procedures were included because of the functional relation between negative arousal (anger) and aggressive behavior.[72, 73] Teaching relaxation to adolescents with anger and disruptive behavior is an effective self-management skill. Further research with BRT and this population is needed. The increasing presence of Board Certified Behavior Analysts in public schools makes the examination of the effect of BRT on the anger and aggressive behavior of children with serious emotional disturbance and conduct disorder much more feasible.

CONCLUSIONS

This chapter reviewed evidence that children and adults with a wide variety of neurodevelopmental disabilities can readily learn relaxation skills using BRT. This training has been associated with improved functioning in fine motor manipulation tasks, short-term memory tests, anxiety and psychiatric symptom ratings, and disruptive outbursts. More research is needed on programs to assist persons with disabilities to incorporate relaxation into their daily lives and to measure effects on activities of daily living. Promising approaches include the development of self-instructional methods, training parents or staff to conduct BRT, and group training in residential facilities. Combining BRT with other self-control methods (e.g., biofeedback, self-instructions) to provide alternatives to dysfunctional behavior in motor, verbal, observational, and visceral modalities needs further exploration.

The BRS has proven useful in measuring relaxation acquisition and maintenance, particularly with persons demonstrating limited verbal capacity. Measurement is an important issue in the evaluation of treatment process and outcome, as discussed in Chapter 3, especially when procedures are modified to meet special participant needs. We urge researchers and clinicians to employ the BRS, a direct observation system. Direct observation requires a precise definition of the target behavior, in contrast to rating scales. A rating system, such as that employed by Lindsay et al.,[20-27] does not allow comparisons across studies conducted by different researchers. A standardized metric, such as the BRS, facilitates communication within the field.

Efficiency and effectiveness are important characteristics of interventions. Because BRT focuses on instruction of overt relaxed behavior, it makes for a more efficient means of teaching relaxation to persons with disabilities. The relaxed behaviors are easily acquired because they are directly observable by both the trainer and participant, and can be immediately reinforced by social or extrinsic consequences. Some supportive data on the superiority of BRT were reported by Lindsay.[20-27] But this should not be taken as a blanket endorsement for BRT over other training methods. The needs and capabilities of each "special" individual should be considered in devising an intervention program, just as they are for anyone else.

The studies detailed in this chapter have provided several insights into a more efficacious use of the protocol with special populations. Discriminating muscle tension (covert motor behavior) and having that event serve as a discriminative stimulus for engaging in the tense-relax exercises of PMR, is difficult to teach with minimally verbal participants. Modeling the relaxed postures of BRT to a person with a disability can significantly increase the likelihood of imitation of the behavior, and, eventually, the relaxed behaviors come under instructional control.[27]

There is also great benefit in providing visual representations of the postures for use by the person when they start to feel upset or are faced with an identified antecedent to aggressive situations. Providing pictures cues of the relaxed behaviors increases the likelihood of maintenance and generalization of relaxation skills in the natural environment and also provides a mechanism to further enhance self-management skills. Other procedures may also be valuable in producing maintenance of skills. Further research is needed in this area.

Adaptations have been made to the BRS that allows for ease of use in residential settings and family members of those with special needs can collect data regarding relaxed behavior. These data can then be incorporated into the overall treatment plan for the person served. By instructing staff to schedule BRT sessions on a daily basis, relaxation training functions as an antecedent control intervention and decreases the effect of aversive motivating operations (stressors). Such training also is necessary for the individual to acquire the skills and use them in the context of events that elicit strong emotional behavior and evoke other maladaptive behaviors. Comprehensive intervention requires that staff and family members be adequately trained in basic prompting and reinforcement procedures to ensure that relaxation self-management skills are performed in the natural environment.

REFERENCES

[1]American Psychiatric Association. (2013). *Diagnostic and statistical manual of mental disorders, 5th Edition*. Washington, D.C.: American Psychiatric Association.

[2]Allen, R., Lindsay, W. R., MacLeod, F., & Smith, A. H. W. (2001), Treatment of women with intellectual disabilities who have been involved with the criminal justice system for reasons of aggression. *Journal of Applied Research in Intellectual Disabilities, 14*, 340–347. doi:10.1046/j.1468-3148.2001.00086.x

[3]Calamari, J. E., Geist, G. O., & Shahbazian, M. J. (1987). Evaluation of multiple component relaxation training with developmentally disabled persons. *Research and Developmental Disabilities, 8*(1), 55–70. https://doi.org/10.1016/0891-4222(87)90040-0

[4]Hanrahan, S. (1998). Practical considerations for working with athletes with disabilities. *The Sport Psychologist, 12*, 346–357. https://doi.org/10.1123/tsp.12.3.346

[5]Harvey, J. R. (1979). The potential of relaxation training for the mentally retarded. *Mental Retardation, 17*, 71–76.

[6]Liberman, R. P., & Corrigan, P. W. (1993). Designing new psychosocial treatments for schizophrenia. *Psychiatry, 56*, 238–248. https://doi.org/10.1080/00332747.1993.11024640

[7]Luiselli, J. K. (1980). Relaxation training with the developmentally disabled: A reappraisal. *Behavior Research with Severe Developmental Disabilities, 1*, 191–213.

[8]McPhali, C. H., & Chamove, A. S. (1989). Relaxation reduces disruption in mentally handicapped adults. *Journal of Mental Deficiency Research, 33* (Pt 5), 399–406. https://doi.org/10.1111/j.1365-2788.1989.tb01494.x

[9]Ortega, D. F. (1978). Relaxation exercises with cerebral palsied adults showing spasticity. *Journal of Applied Behavior Analysis, 11*, 447–451. https://doi.org/10.1901/jaba.1978.11-447

[10]Reiss, S. (1982). Psychopathology and mental retardation: A survey of a developmental disabilities mental health program. *Mental Retardation, 20*, 128–132.

[11]Reiss, S., Levitan, G. W., & McNally, R. J. (1982). Emotionally disturbed mentally retarded people: An underserved population. *American Psychologist, 37*, 361–367. https://doi.org/10.1037/0003-066X.37.4.361

[12]Myin-Germeys, I., & Van os, J. (2007). Stress-reactivity in psychosis: Evidence for an affective pathway to psychosis. *Clinical Psychology Review, 27*(4), 409–424. https://doi.org/10.1016/j.cpr.2006.09.005

[13]Sturmey, P. (2004), Cognitive therapy with people with intellectual disabilities: a selective review and critique. *Clinical Psychology and Psychotherapy, 11*, 222–232. doi:10.1002/cpp.409

[14]Whitaker, S., & Read, S. (2006), The prevalence of psychiatric disorders among people with intellectual disabilities: An analysis of the literature. *Journal of Applied Research in Intellectual Disabilities, 19*, 330–345. doi:10.1111/j.1468-3148.2006.00293.

[15]Taylor, J. L. (2009). Treatment of anger and aggression for offenders with intellectual disabilities in secure settings. In R. Didden & X. Moonen (Eds.), *Met het oog op behandeling.* (pp. 9–14). Amersfoort, The Netherlands: Bergdrukkerij.

[16]Singh, N. N., Lancioni, G. E., Winton, A. S. W., Singh, A. N., Adkins, A. D., & Singh. J. (2008). Clinical and benefit-cost outcomes of teaching a mindfulness-based treatment

of anger and aggression procedure to adult offenders with intellectual disabilities. *Behavior Modification, 32,* 622–637. https://doi.org/10.1177/0145445508315854

[17]McGimpsey, B. A. (1982). *Behavioral relaxation training and assessment with developmentally disabled adults.* Unpublished master's thesis, Southern Illinois University at Carbondale.

[18]Paclawski, T R., & Yoo, J. H. (2006). Behavioral relaxation training (BRT) Facilitating acquisition in individuals with developmental disabilities. *The NADD Bulletin, 9,* 13–17.

[19]Keisel, K. B., Lutzker, J. R., & Campbell, R. V. (1989). Behavioral relaxation training to reduce hyperventilation and seizures in a profoundly retarded epileptic child. *Journal of the Multihandicapped Person, 2*(3), 179–190. https://doi.org/10.1007/BF01100089

[20]Lindsay, W. R., Allan, R., Parry, C., Macleod, F., Cottrell, J., Overend, H., & Smith, A. H. W. (2004). Anger and aggression in people with intellectual disabilities: treatment and follow-up of consecutive referrals and a waiting list comparison. *Clinical Psychology & Psychotherapy, 11,* 255–264. https://doi.org/10.1002/cpp.415

[21]Lindsay, W.R., Overend, H, Allan, R., Williams, C., & Black, L. (1998). Using specific approaches for individual problems in the management of anger and aggression. *British Journal of Learning Disabilities, 26*(2), 44–50. https://doi.org/10.1111/j.1468-3156.1998.tb00047.x

[22]Lindsay, W. R., Baty, F. J., Michie, A. M., & Richardson, I. (1989). A comparison of anxiety treatments with adults who have moderate and severe mental retardation. *Research in Developmental Disabilities, 10*(2), 129–140. https://doi.org/10.1016/0891-4222(89)90002-4

[23]Lindsay, W. R., Richardson, I., & Michie, A. M. (1989). Short-term generalized effects of relaxation training on adults with moderate and severe mental handicaps. *Journal of Applied Research in Intellectual Disabilities, 2,* 197–206. https://doi.org/10.1111/j.1468-3148.1989.tb00027.x

[24]Lindsay, W. R., & Morrison, F. M. (1996). The effects of behavioral relaxation on cognitive performance in adults with severe intellectual disabilities. *Journal of Intellectual Disability Research, 40,* 285–290. https://doi.org/10.1111/j.1365-2788.1996.tb00632.x

[25]Lindsay, W. R., & Baty, F. J. (1986a). Abbreviated progressive relaxation: Its use with adults who are mentally handicapped. *Mental Handicap, 14,* 123–126. https://doi.org/10.1111/j.1468-3156.1986.tb00362.x

[26]Lindsay, W. R., & Baty, F. J. (1986b). Behavioral relaxation training: Explorations with adults who are mentally handicapped. Mental Handicap, 14, 160–162. https://doi.org/10.1111/j.1468-3156.1986.tb00373.x

[27]Lindsay, W. R., & Baty, F. J., Michie, A., & Heap, I. (1994). The effects of cue control relaxation on adults with severe mental retardation. Research in Developmental Disabilities, 15, 425–437. https://doi.org/10.1016/0891-4222(94)90027-2

[28]Burgio, L. D., Whitman, T. L., & Johnson, M. R. (1980). A self-instructional package for increasing attending behavior in educable mentally retarded children. *Journal of Applied Behavior Analysis, 13*(3), 443–459. https://doi.org/10.1901/jaba.1980.13-443

[29]Lundervold, D. A. (1986). The effects of behavioral relaxation and self-instruction training: A case study. *Rehabilitation Counseling Bulletin, 30*(2), 124–128.

[30]van Steensel, F. J. A. Bogels, S. M., & Perrin, S. (2011). Anxiety disorders in children and adolescents with autistic spectrum disorder: A meta-analysis. *Clinical Child and Family Psychology Review, 14*, 302–317. https://doi.org/10.1007/s10567-011-0097-0

[31]White, S. W., Oswald, D., Ollendick, T., & Scahill, L. (2009). Anxiety in children and adolescents with autism spectrum disorders. *Clinical Psychology Review, 29*(3), 216–229. doi:10.1016/j.cpr.2009.01.003.

[32]Simonoff, E., Pickles, A., Charman, T., Chandler, S., Loucas, T., & Baird, G. (2008). Psychiatric disorders in children with autism spectrum disorders: Prevalence, comorbidity, and associated factors in a population-derived sample. *Journal of the American Academy of Child & Adolescent Psychiatry, 47*, 921–929. https://doi.org/10.1097/CHI.0b013e318179964f

[33]Costello, J. E., Egger, H. J., & Angold, A. (2005). The developmental epidemiology of anxiety disorders: Phenomenology, prevalence, and comorbidity. *Child and Adolescent Psychiatric Clinics of North America, 14*, 631–648. https://doi.org/10.1016/j.chc.2005.06.003

[34]Cervantes, P., & Matson, J. L. (2015). Comorbid symptomology in adults with autism spectrum disorder and intellectual disability. *Journal of Autism and Developmental Disorders, 45*, 3961–3970. https://doi.org/10.1007/s10803-015-2553-z

[35]Chalfant, A. M., Rapee, R., & Carroll, L. (2007). Treating anxiety disorders in children with high functioning autism spectrum disorders: A controlled trial. *Journal of Autism and Developmental Disorders, 37*(10), 1842. https://doi.org/10.1007/s10803-006-0318-4

[36]Reaven, J., Blakeley-Smith, A., Culhane-Shelburne, K., & Hepburn, S. (2012). Group cognitive behavior therapy for children with high-functioning autism spectrum disorders and anxiety: A randomized trial. *Journal of Child Psychology and Psychiatry, 53*(4), 410–419. https://doi.org/10.1111/j.1469-7610.2011.02486.x

[37]Storch, E. A., Arnold, E. B., Lewin, A. B., Nadeau, J. M., Jones, A. M., De Nadai, A. S. Mutch, M., Selles, R. R., Ung, D., & Murphy, T. K. (2013). The effect of cognitive-behavioral therapy versus treatment as usual for anxiety in children with autism spectrum disorders: A randomized, controlled trial. *Journal of the American Academy of Child & Adolescent Psychiatry, 52*(2), 132–142. https://doi.org/10.1016/j.jaac.2012.11.007

[38]Sukhodolsky, D. G., Bloch, M. H., Panza, K.E., & Reichow, B. (2013). Cognitive-behavioral therapy for anxiety in children with high-functioning autism: A meta-analysis. *Pediatrics*. 2013 Nov; 132(5): e1341–e1350. https://doi.org/10.1542/peds.2013-1193

[39]Bechtler, J. (2011). *Reduction of anxiety in college students with Asperger's disorder using behavioral relaxation training.* (2011). Theses and Dissertations. http://rdw.rowan.edu/etd/82?utm_source=rdw.rowan.edu%2Fetd%2F82&utm_medium=PDF&utm_campaign=PDFCoverPages

[40]Lodge, D. J., & Grace, A. A. (2011). Developmental pathology, dopamine, stress and schizophrenia. *International Journal of Developmental Neuroscience, 29*, 207–213. https://doi.org/10.1016/j.ijdevneu.2010.08.002

[41]van Winkel, R., Stefanis, N. C., & Myin-Germeys, I. (2008). Psychosocial stress and psychosis. A review of the neurobiological mechanisms and the evidence for

gene-stress interaction. *Schizophrinia Bulletin, 34*(6):1095–105. doi: 10.1093/schbul/sbn101

[42]Phillips, L. J., Francey, S. M., Edwards, J., & McMurray, N. (2007). Stress and psychosis: Towards the development of new models of investigation. *Clinical Psychology Review, 27*(3), 307–317. https://doi.org/10.1016/j.cpr.2006.10.003

[43]Howes, O. D., McCutcheon, R., Owen, M. J., & Murray, R. M. (2017). The role of genes, stress, and dopamine in the development of schizophrenia. *Biological Psychiatry, 81*(1):9–20. doi: 10.1016/j.biopsych.2016.07.014

[44]Gajsak, L. R., Gelemanovic, A., Kuzman, M. R., & Puljak, L. (2017). Impact of stress response in development of first-episode psychosis in schizophrenia: An overview of systematic reviews. *Psychiatra Danubia, 29*(1), 14–23. https://doi.org/10.24869/psyd.2017.14

[45]Acosta, F. X., Yamamoto, J., & Wilcox, S. A. (1978). Application of electromyographic feedback to the relaxation training of schizophrenic, neurotic, and tension headache participants. *Journal of Consulting and Clinical Psychology, 46*, 383–384. https://doi.org/10.1037/0022-006X.46.2.383

[46]Pharr, O. M., & Coursey, R. D. (1989). The use and utility of EMG biofeedback with chronic schizophrenic participants. *Biofeedback and Self-Regulation, 14*, 229–245. https://doi.org/10.1007/BF01000096

[47]Rickard, H. C., Collier, J. R., McCoy, A. D., Crist, D. A., & Weinberger, M. B. (1993). Relaxation training for psychiatric in participants. *Psychological Reports, 72*, 1267–1274. https://doi.org/10.2466/pr0.1993.72.3c.1267

[48]Chen, W., Chu, H., Lu, R., Chou, Y., Chen, C., Chang, Y., O'Brien, A.P., & Chou, K. (2009). Efficacy of progressive muscle relaxation training in reducing anxiety in participants with acute schizophrenia. *Complementary and Alternative Medicine, 18*(15), 218–2196. https://doi.org/10.1111/j.1365-2702.2008.02773.x

[49]Vancampfort, D., Correll, C. U., Scheewe, T. W., Probst, M., De Herdt, A., Knapen, J., & De Hert, M. (2012). Progressive muscle relaxation in persons with schizophrenia: a systematic review of randomized controlled trials. *Clinical Rehabilitation, 27*(4), 291–298. https://doi.org/10.1177/0269215512455531

[50]Noe, S. R. (1997). *Behavioral relaxation training to reduce autonomic hyperarousal in individuals with schizophrenia*. Unpublished doctoral dissertation, Southern Illinois University at Carbondale.

[51]Spielberger, C. D. (1983). *State-Trait Anxiety Inventory*. Odessa, FL: Psychological Assessment Resources.

[52]Overall, J. E., & Gorham, D. R. (1962). The brief psychiatric rating scale. *Psychological Reports, 10*, 799–812. https://doi.org/10.2466/pr0.1962.10.3.799

[53]Carbray, J. A. (2018). Attention-Deficit/Hyperactivity Disorder in children and adolescents. *Journal of Psychosocial Nursing and Mental Health Services, 56*(12), 7–10. doi: 10.3928/02793695-20181112-02.

[54]Faraone, S. V., & Biederman, J. (2005). What is the prevalence of adult ADHD? Results of a population screen of 966 adults. *Journal of Attention Disorders, 9*, 384–391. https://doi.org/10.1177/1087054705281478

[55]Biederman, J., Wilens, T., Mick, E. et al. (1997). Is ADHD a risk factor for psychoactive substance use disorders? Findings from a four-year prospective follow-

up study. *Journal of the American Academy of Child and Adolescent Psychiatry, 36,* 21–29. https://doi.org/10.1097/00004583-199701000-00013

[56]Arias, A. J., Gelernter, J., Chan, G., Weiss, R. D., Brady, K. T., Farrer, L., & Kranzler, H. R. (2008). Correlates of co-occurring ADHD in drug-dependent Participants: Prevalence and features of substance dependence and psychiatric disorders. *Addictive Behaviors, 33,* 1199–1207. https://doi.org/10.1016/j.addbeh.2008.05.003

[57]Mash, E. J., & Johnston, C. (1983). Parental perceptions of child behavior problems, parenting self-esteem, and mothers' reported stress in younger and older hyperactive and normal children. *Journal of Consulting and Clinical Psychology, 51,* 86–99. https://doi.org/10.1037/0022-006X.51.1.86

[58]Murphy, K. R., & Barkley, R. A. (1996). Parents of children with attention deficit/hyperactivity disorder: psychological and attentional impairment. *American Journal of Orthopsychiatry, 66,* 93–102. https://doi.org/10.1037/h0080159

[59]Ben-Naim. S., Gill, N., Laslo-Roth, R., & Einav, M. (2018). Parental stress and parental self-efficacy as mediators of the association between children's ADHD and marital satisfaction. *Journal of Attention Disorder,* In press. https://doi.org/10.1177/1087054718784659

[60]Cowles, B. J. (2009). Update on the management of attention-deficit/hyperactivity disorder in children and adults: Participant considerations and the role of lisdexamfetamine. *Therapeutics and Clinical Risk Management, 5,* 943–48. https://doi.org/10.2147/TCRM.S6733

[61]Handen, B. L., Feldman, H., Gosling, A., Breaux A. M., & McCauliffe, S. (1991). Adverse side effects of methylphenidate among mentally retarded children with ADHD. *Journal of the American Academy of Child and Adolescent Psychiatry, 30*(2), 241–245. https://doi.org/10.1097/00004583-199103000-00012

[62]Martinez-Raga, J., Knecht, C., Szerman, N., & Martinez, M. I. (2013). Risk of serious cardiovascular problems with medications for attention-deficit hyperactivity disorder. *Central Nervous System Drugs, 27*(1), 15–30. doi: 10.1007/s40263-012-0019

[63]Raymer, R. H., & Poppen, R. (1985). Behavioral relaxation training with hyperactive children. *Journal of Behavior Therapy and Experimental Psychiatry, 16,* 309–316. https://doi.org/10.1016/0005-7916(85)90005-9

[64]Barkley, R. A. (1981). *Hyperactive children: A handbook for diagnosis and treatment.* New York: Guilford.

[65]Goyette, C. H., Conners, C. K., & Ulrich, R. F. (1978). Normative data on revised Conners parent and teacher rating scales. *Journal of Abnormal Child Psychology, 6,* 221–236. https://doi.org/10.1007/BF00919127

[66]Donney, V. K., & Poppen, R. (1989). Teaching parents to conduct behavioral relaxation training with their hyperactive children. *Journal of Behavior Therapy and Experimental Psychiatry, 20,* 319–325. https://doi.org/10.1016/0005-7916(89)90063-3

[67]Friedman, R. M., & Kutash, K. (1986). *Mad, bad, sad, can't add. Florida Adolescent and Child Treatment Study.* Tampa: Florida Mental Health Institute.

[68]Capaldi, D. M., & Dishion, T. J. (1993). *The relation of conduct problems and depressive symptoms to growth in substance use in adolescent boys.* Eugene OR: Social Learning Center.

[69]Gilliam, J. E., & Scott, B. K. (1987). The behaviorally disordered offender. In R. Rutherford, C. Nelson, & B. Wolford (Eds.), *Special education in correctional education.* Columbus, OH: Merrill.

[70]Baum, J., G., Clark, H. B., McCarthy, W., Sandler, J., & Carpenter, R. (1986). An analysis of the acquisition and generalization of socials skills in troubled youth: Combining social skills, cognitive self-talk and relaxation procedures. *Child and Family Behavior Therapy, 8,* 1–27. https://doi.org/10.1300/J019v08n04_01

[71]Schilling, D. J., & Poppen, R. (1983). Behavioral relaxation training and assessment. *Journal of Experimental Psychiatry and Behavior Therapy, 14,* 99–107. https://doi.org/10.1016/0005-7916(83)90027-7

[72]Novaco, R. W. (1976). Treatment of chronic anger through cognitive and relaxation controls. *Journal of Consulting and Clinical Psychology, 44,* 681. https://doi.org/10.1037/0022-006X.44.4.681

[73]Novaco, R. W. (1979). *Cognitive-behavioral interventions. Theory, research and procedures.* NY: Academic Press.

Supplement
Behavior Analyst Certification Board 5th Edition Task List

A. Philosophical Underpinnings
A-1   Identify the goals of behavior analysis as a science (i.e., description, prediction, control).

A-2   Explain the philosophical assumptions underlying the science of behavior analysis (e.g., selectionism, determinism, empiricism, parsimony, pragmatism).

A-3   Describe and explain behavior from the perspective of radical behaviorism.

A-4   Distinguish among behaviorism, the experimental analysis of behavior, applied behavior analysis, and professional practice guided by the science of behavior analysis.

A-5   Describe and define the dimensions of applied behavior analysis (Baer, Wolf, & Risley, (1968).

B. Concepts and Principles
B-1   Define and provide examples of behavior, response, and response class.

B-2   Define and provide examples of stimulus and stimulus class.

B-3   Define and provide examples of respondent and operant conditioning.

B-4   Define and provide examples of positive and negative reinforcement contingencies.

B-5   Define and provide examples of schedules of reinforcement.

B-10   Define and provide examples of stimulus control.

C. Measurement, Data Display, and Interpretation
C-1   Establish operational definitions of behavior.

C-2   Distinguish among direct, indirect, and product measures of behavior.

C-3   Measure occurrence (e.g., frequency, rate, percentage).

C-5   Measure form and strength of behavior (e.g., topography, magnitude).

C-6   Measure trials to criterion.

C-7   Design and implement sampling procedures (i.e., interval recording, time sampling).

C-8   Evaluate the validity and reliability of measurement procedures.

C-9 Select a measurement system to obtain representative data given the dimensions of behavior and the logistics of observing and recording.
C-10 Graph data to communicate relevant quantitative relations (e.g., equal-interval graphs, bar graphs, cumulative records).
C-11 Interpret graphed data.

D. Experimental Design
D-1 Distinguish between dependent and independent variables.
D-5 Use single-subject experimental designs (e.g., reversal, multiple baseline, multielement, changing criterion).

G. Behavior-Change Procedures
G-1 Use positive and negative reinforcement procedures to strengthen behavior.
G-5 Use modeling and imitation training.
G-6 Use instructions and rules.
G-9 Use discrete-trial, free-operant, and naturalistic teaching arrangements.
G-14 Use reinforcement procedures to weaken behavior (e.g., DRA, FCT, DRO, DRL, NCR).
G-17 Use token economies.
G-20 Use self-management strategies.

H. Selecting and Implementing Interventions
H-1 State intervention goals in observable and measurable terms.
H-4 When a target behavior is to be decreased, select an acceptable alternative behavior to be established or increased.
H-6 Monitor client progress and treatment integrity.
H-7 Make data-based decisions about the effectiveness of the intervention and the need for treatment revision.
H-9 Collaborate with others who support and/or provide services to clients.

I. Personnel Supervision and Management
I-4 Train personnel to competently perform assessment and intervention procedures.

Chapter 6
Pain and Anxiety Disorders

Chronic pain and anxiety impact significant numbers of people across the lifespan on a daily basis. Current population-based estimates of chronic pain in the United States range from 11 to 40 percent,[1] and according to the National Comorbidity Survey Replication study, 18 percent of Americans suffer from an anxiety disorder.[2] Analgesic and anxiolytic medication is by far the primary treatment mode for these disorders, but medications often do not provide complete relief and may be associated with unwanted side-effects as well as dependency issues. Stress is a significant factor in pain and anxiety problems and often a vicious circle arises, in which pain or anxiety further increase the demands with which the individual is trying to cope. Behavioral interventions offer adaptive ways to deal with stress, pain, and anxiety disorders. This chapter reviews behavioral interventions that include BRT.

PAIN DISORDERS

Self-management approaches to chronic pain recognize the important relationships among perceived pain, physiological arousal, and negative emotions and cognition (visceral and verbal behavior). Stress can arise from the experience of pain and dealing with limitations imposed by pain. This stress can exacerbate pain, resulting in a vicious circle leading to severe disability, emotional dysfunction, and dysfunctional rule-governed behavior. Thus, relaxation training is often employed as a component of many pain management programs to reduce arousal. This section describes pain-management programs that include BRT.

Headache

Headaches are extremely common; estimates are that nearly half the adult population has experienced at least one in the past year. They vary widely in frequency and intensity. A *headache disorder* is recognized when they recur to such an extent so as to interfere with a person's ability to function in social or employment settings. Cumulatively, society suffers tremendous loss in terms of costs of treatment and diminished productivity.

The two most frequent types of headache are *migraine* and *tension*. Migraine symptoms typically include pain on one side of the head (the Latin *hemi crania* or half head); sharp, stabbing or throbbing pain; exacerbated by light, noise, or physical activity; preceded or accompanied by nausea; preceded by visual or other sensory anomalies called an *aura*. Tension headache pain is experienced as an ache or tightness encircling the skull, sometimes including the back of the neck. Some people experience *mixed* headache, with symptoms of both migraine and tension.

There are many other types of headache, some of which are secondary to severe disorders, such as brain tumor. No one should undertake intervention with a headache participant without a medical examination and referral.[3]

The contemporary conceptualization of migraine is as a biobehavioral disorder involving vascular, neurologic, multiple brain structures, and genetic and environmental stress factors.[4] The rationale for employing relaxation in the treatment of migraine and tension headache has generally followed a stress model, focusing on motor and visceral responses to stressful life events. Relaxation, according to this model, serves as a prophylactic, preventing or reversing the physiological arousal.

"CLASSIC" MIGRAINE. Edward B. Blanchard found that a program of progressive relaxation and imagery resulted in clinically significant headache reduction for approximately 26 percent of migraine sufferers, whereas an added program of thermal biofeedback essentially doubled the success rate.[5]

This case employed Blanchard's migraine protocol but substituted BRT for PMR. Miss B was a 34-year-old woman, a college graduate employed in a managerial position, with a ten-year history of headache. She was diagnosed by a neurologist as "classic migraine" and met Blanchard's research criteria for frequency and intensity. Miss B also had a diagnosis of bipolar disorder of six years duration which was controlled by lithium. She reported few current depressive symptoms and her score on the Beck Depression Inventory was in the normal range throughout the treatment program.

The Headache Diary, in which she rated her headache on a 6-point scale (0 = *no headache,* 3 = *moderate headache, pain is noticeably present,* 5 = *extremely intense headache, incapacitated*), was completed four times daily. A weekly Headache Index was computed by summing all scores and dividing by seven, thus incorporating both frequency and intensity. She also recorded any headache medications taken and a potency score was calculated. Measurement occurred throughout baseline treatment and follow up.

During each session, frontalis and cervical trapezius EMG levels, finger temperature, and the BRS were measured in five-minute pre- and post-training observation periods. Self-report of relaxation was measured after each observation period. Miss B was given a stress rationale and was told that relaxation would provide her with a means by which she could control her arousal, particularly her vascular reactions. A three-phase stepped-care treatment program, with six sessions per phase, was planned. The phases were BRT, thermal biofeedback, and stress identification and problem solving. A four-week break between each phase was scheduled to assess its effects before going on to the next one. But as it turned out, headache frequency was reduced to such an extent in the first (BRT) phase that the other two phases were not implemented.

Two sessions of reclined BRT were provided, followed by diaphragmatic breathing training during BRT. The next two sessions were devoted to Upright Relaxation Training (URT) and diaphragmatic breathing. The use of diaphragmatic breathing and mini-relaxation throughout the day was emphasized as an immediate tool to counteract arousal and maintain calmness.

Consistent with earlier research, the relaxed behaviors were acquired very rapidly. The BRS and self-report scores were moderately related (Pearson $r = .59$, $p < .05$). Miss B reached 92 percent relaxed by the end of the second session and reported she was "deeply and completely relaxed." Diaphragmatic breathing training increased unrelaxed behavior and self-reported tension, but by the end of the next session scores again were low. Both BRS and self-report scores were elevated at the start of URT in the fifth session but decreased with training. Reclined relaxed behavior was maintained at the seventh session.

Frontalis and cervical EMG levels were quite variable and not correlated with each other or with other measures. Miss B's pre-training finger temperatures started in the mid-90s, a ceiling that made further increases unlikely. Temperatures often declined during BRT and diaphragmatic breathing training. However, during URT, her temperatures were high and stable, and remained high at post-training assessment. Overall, her temperature was correlated with BRS scores (Pearson $r = .67$, $p < .05$).

Weekly headache index scores declined markedly. During baseline, Ms. B experienced at least one headache per week, which she said was her usual rate. She reported one major headache the second week of training, and one in the second week of the post-training period, but otherwise was headache free. It should be noted that this was during the holiday period, which was a generally stressful time for her. Using Blanchard's formula for calculating treatment outcome, Miss B experienced 76 percent reduction in headache, well above the 50 percent reduction considered a "success."[5] Her medication index score also showed a clinically significant reduction.

During the first six weeks of the six-month follow-up, she reported one severe headache which she said was the first she'd experienced since treatment ended. She reported, however, when a headache did occur, it seemed more intense, but noted that this may have been due to her not being as "used to" the pain.

At the six-month follow-up interview, Miss B stated that she did not set aside time to practice. But she reported being more aware of her postures and using deep breathing and mini-relaxation sessions during the day, and that she was able to relax when becoming "uptight." She also reported that she had started jogging, and felt that this also contributed to her remaining headache free.

MIXED HEADACHE IN AN INDIVIDUAL WITH INTELLECTUAL DISABILITY. According to Walsh and colleagues,[6] individuals with intellectual disabilities (ID) have a high incidence of chronic pain that results in significant limitations in daily functioning. Reports of educating practitioners about pain assessment among individuals with ID has grown,[7-9] while at the same time, the literature describing non-medical pain management remains very sparse.[10-13] McGuire and colleagues[10] conclude that persons with ID have an increased risk of chronic pain but are under-served, especially those with impaired communication ability.

Michultka, Poppen, and Blanchard[14] reported one of the few cases of intervention for chronic pain in a person with ID. Ben, a 29-year old male with severe intellectual disabilities (Stanford-Binet IQ < 30), related to anoxia at birth, lived at a community group care home. He was minimally verbal, communicating with one or two-word requests, and sometimes could follow simple instructions. Ben had been diagnosed with both classic migraine and tension headache for ten years. He had been taught to indicate the type of headache to staff members, who could then administer appropriate analgesic medication.

Training was conducted intermittently for a total of twenty sessions over a four-month period. Regular scheduling was precluded by the participant's frequent episodes of violent behavior, resulting in canceled appointments. In an initial session, the participant was asked to relax for a 30-minute period. For the next ten sessions, BRT acquisition training was administered as described previously for special populations. Postures were taught in a cumulative fashion, with successive time requirements of 5, 10, 30, and 60 seconds for each. Contingent on maintaining the relaxed posture at criterion level, Ben received verbal praise. Scheduled breaks were taken midway through each session, at which time Ben had a small glass of iced tea, a favorite drink.

After learning all ten behaviors, Ben received nine proficiency training sessions. He was taught to demonstrate each of the relaxed behaviors sequentially and was then given the verbal cue "relax" as a signal to do all of them together. Throughout the proficiency training process Ben was given periodic corrective feedback and verbal praise as he practiced. After he reached the criterion on proficiency training, a three-month follow-up visit was scheduled. He was encouraged by staff to practice BRT on his own, but no formal records were kept.

The BRS was scored for three five-minute intervals during the first baseline session and at the conclusion of each training session. Frequency of headache complaints and amount of medication consumption were recorded routinely by the direct care staff. Headache and medication records were available for the four months preceding training and for two months afterwards. No records were available concerning his aggressive behavior.

Ten and nine sessions, respectively, were required for acquisition and proficiency training to reach a criterion of at least 80 percent relaxed over three consecutive sessions. Acquisition training was slowed by the irregular schedule; the participant often appeared to forget previously trained behavior after a lapse of several days or weeks. Ben demonstrated 90 percent relaxed behaviors at a three-month follow-up.

Monthly headache frequency averaged about seven per month for the four months preceding training. Frequency increased to about twelve per month during the first two months of BRT and then fell precipitously to about three per month during the last two months of training, remaining at this level for two months following training. Medication consumption decreased along with headache frequency. Informal follow-up at three months with a guardian, with whom the participant had gone to live, revealed that headaches were infrequent and the use of medication for tension headache had been discontinued.

TENSION HEADACHE. Betty,[15] a 21-year-old woman, employed as a nurse, reported she had experienced tension headaches since childhood. She estimated current frequency ranging from three to eight per month, with severity rated from mild to severe. A recent neurological exam ruled out other factors.

Betty rated her headache intensity on a 0 to 5 scale and recorded its duration, producing a daily headache score, for two weeks of baseline. Two BRT sessions took place in her home during week three, following baseline. Session duration, spacing, and BRS scores were not reported, though it's implied she became proficient in relaxing. Betty was asked to practice relaxation for 20 minutes twice a day and whenever she felt stressed. During the fourth week, EMG biofeedback from her frontalis muscles was added to BRT for two sessions. Two final sessions of BRT alone occurred in week five. Thereafter, she recorded headaches for a six-month follow-up period.

Betty reported headaches, of varying duration and intensity, on 11 of 14 days during baseline. Her headache score fell to zero during the first BRT week; one severe headache during the week of BRT+EMG, and zero again during the final BRT week. In the follow-up period, Betty reported one headache during the first and third months, and a very severe headache lasting five days, during month four. Months two, five, and six were headache free.

Frontalis EMG levels were recorded on three separate occasions during baseline, and during the BRT and biofeedback sessions. It was noted that EMG was elevated on the baseline day Betty was experiencing headache, and declined from baseline resting levels during BRT. Biofeedback resulted in no greater decrease in frontalis tension than BRT alone and probably was irrelevant for the headache reductions that occurred.

NEUROFACIAL PAIN. Mrs. C[16] was a 47-year-old woman with two children and a graduate degree in education. She was very active in community and church affairs. Six months prior to the initial contact, she had been diagnosed with atypical neurofacial pain in the maxillary region of the trigeminal nerve following three months of medical treatment for a sinus infection. She took large doses of Nortriptoline and Motrin daily but reported no relief. A maxillary nerve block provided short-term pain relief, and nerve ablation surgery was offered as a treatment option. However, her referring physician suggested that she try behavioral treatment before more invasive procedures.

A structured interview for chronic/recurrent pain and an EMG muscle scan of facial and neck muscles was administered. Mrs. C monitored pain four times daily using a modification of the Blanchard Headache Diary described previously. She reported almost continuous pain on the right side of her face, described as burning and throbbing, sometimes accompanied by blurred vision, varying from "moderate" to "incapacitating." The muscle scan revealed asymmetrically high readings in the right masseter, sternocleidomastoid, and cervical trapezius. Mrs. C reported clenching her jaw when upset. She reported that depression, irritability, and dread accompanied severe pain episodes and that pain interfered with her family and volunteer duties. She reported that pain was exacerbated by worry, tension, and anger, noting there was a strong relationship between stress and pain. Life stressors, in addition to pain, included her husband's health and professional problems, severe illness of family members, demands of her volunteer commitments, and the job of raising two active sons.

Weekly 50-minute sessions were conducted. Approximately 15 minutes were devoted to BRT, with the balance spent in discussing how to implement relaxation in her daily life. After a baseline session, in which she relaxed in her usual way, BRT in the reclined position was conducted for two sessions, followed by Upright BRT for three sessions. Each session concluded with a five-minute observation period for BRS scoring and monitoring masseter EMG activity. She was instructed to practice relaxation daily. A five-step *mini-relaxation program* was devised: stop and sit, close eyes, deep inhale, drop jaw, and exhale. These comprised a set of self-instructions that she employed throughout her heavily scheduled day. She agreed to use transitions between activities as a cue to engage in mini-relaxation. A follow-up session employing URT was conducted two months after training.

Mrs. C's baseline BRS was a surprising 86 percent relaxed. With training, she attained BRS scores of about 97 percent. BRS after her first upright session dropped to 92 percent but subsequently increased to 100 percent relaxed for the remainder of training and follow-up. Masseter EMG activity was fairly high during baseline but decreased by 50 percent during reclined BRT and by another 50 percent during UBRT. EMG levels increased slightly during mini-relaxation practice but returned to very low levels at follow-up.

Mrs. C's daily pain ratings averaged around 3 (moderate) during baseline and did not change appreciably during reclined BRT. Her pain ratings declined to as low as 1 with UBRT and mini-relaxation, but she experienced increased pain during two periods in which her sister and mother-in-law were seriously ill and there were several weeks with no training. She found the mini-relaxation breaks very helpful and reported using them ten to fifteen times daily. By follow-up, her pain ratings were about one-tenth of baseline levels, and she reported large decreases in use of pain medication.

Fibromyalgia

Fibromyalgia (FM) is one of the most common disorders treated at rheumatology clinics, with five percent of women and approximately two percent of men estimated to have FM.[17] A number of physiological mechanisms associated with fibromyalgia and pain dysregulation have been described.[18,19] FM symptoms are diverse and affect different organ and sensory systems, including chronic, diffuse musculoskeletal pain, "tender points" throughout the body, fatigue and sleep disturbance.[20-21] Participants also complain of depression, memory problems and "fibro fog."[21] Needless to say, FM participants are high utilizers of healthcare services. Stress has been reported to exacerbate FM symptoms, in part due to a hypothesized dysregulation of the autonomic nervous system.[19]

To gain a better understanding of interbehavioral dependences and pain behavior, measurement has increasingly focused on the motor, emotional and verbal components of pain behavior. Pain anxiety[22,23] is a response class comprised of emotional, verbal, physiological sensations (responses), and escape/avoidance behavior, each of which has operant and respondent functions depending on context.[24] Past behavior analytic research found to be effective for the treatment of chronic pain has focused on altering the frequency of overt pain behaviors.[25,26] Nonetheless, it has been argued that a pure overt-behavior-focused intervention is inadequate in the treatment of chronic pain.[27]

Behavior analytic interventions for pain management are designed to lessen the aversiveness of pain, thus increasing the likelihood that healthy, non-pain behavior will be more likely to occur. An explicit behavioral activation approach has been proven effective with depression[28,29] with which chronic pain shares much in common. The following two case studies describe Behavioral Activation Treatment for Pain (BAT-P), with BRT serving as a major component.[30,31]

FIBROMYALGIA AND DEPRESSION. ZB was a 43-year-old woman with an 11-year history of fibromyalgia-related pain. She also suffered from essential tremor, migraine headache, and sub-clinical irritable bowel syndrome. ZB also struggled with depression and social phobia. ZB was taking Vicodin 375 mg twice per day; Ibuprofen 800 mg four to six times a day, and Xanax as needed. She was stabilized on the medication before beginning the behavioral intervention.

Measures of Pain Interference Rating (PIR) were taken daily at home using a 10-cm visual analog scale. Pain anxiety was measured by the Pain Anxiety Symptom Score (PASS)[23] and depression by the Geriatric Depression Scale–Short Form (GDS-15).[32] These two measures, along with relaxed behavior (BRS), were assessed every session. ZB also was asked to record her use of prescription pain medications each day. The medication and dosage was used to calculate the Medication Index Score, described earlier. Duration of "healthy up-time behavior" was also recorded each day.

The goal of BAT-P is based on the matching law:[33] increasing the density of reinforcement for overt healthy behavior, while minimizing reinforcement for unhealthy behavior. For example, engaging in relaxed behavior lessened the aversiveness of pain (negative reinforcement), while identifying and engaging in valued activities increased the density of positive reinforcement. The components of BAT-P were BRT, visual feedback, shaping performance of valued up-time activities, and praise. Visual feedback was provided each session related to PIR, depression, and BRS scores. Activity-relaxation cycles were employed to establish a rich schedule of reinforcement for healthy behavior.

Sessions were conducted once per week for about an hour. Baseline measures of PIR, depression, and pain anxiety were obtained. ZB was severely depressed, based on the GDS-15, with moderate to severe pain anxiety on the PASS. Her mean PIR score for the week was 6.25 on a 10-cm scale. Due to the severity of ZB's depression, a controlled clinical approach to assessment and intervention was employed, using a repeated pre-post single-subject research design. Each session began with collecting the homework, assessment of relaxation skills, and proceeding to review, discussion, and feedback regarding homework, and observing within-session relaxation skills.

Session one focused on obtaining informed consent, gathering ZB's clinical history, and establishing the treatment schedule. At the second session, baseline assessment of reclined relaxed behavior was obtained. A biobehavioral conceptualization of chronic pain was then provided; this described physical deconditioning, loss of reinforcers, and avoidance behavior related to pain. Emphasis was placed on self-management of pain and healthy living. Six sessions of Reclined and nine sessions of Upright BRT were conducted. Each training session lasted 15 to 20 minutes, followed by a five-minute post-training observation of relaxed behavior. Interobserver agreement on relaxed behavior was obtained on 28 percent of the sessions (M=84%).

Following the initial assessment, ZB was instructed to relax every two hours at home, following a 15–5 activity-relaxation cycle (15 minutes of up time, five minutes of reclined/upright relaxation), and completion of the PIR and medication usage scales at the end of each day. At the sixth session, Upright BRT was initiated and ZB was instructed in the use of the Valued Behavior Checklist to identify reinforcers that she could come in contact with through scheduling the activity during the day. A list of valued activities was made for each day. Instructions regarding relaxation and activity-relaxation cycles remained the same.

A three-month follow-up assessment of reclined and upright relaxed behavior was conducted. Shortly before this visit, ZB had been mailed the PIR, daily up-time and medication recording form. Measures of depression and pain anxiety were also obtained at the follow-up visit.

Figure 6.1 shows pre- and post-training BRS scores for Reclined and Upright BRT sessions. Relatively low levels of relaxed behaviors were observed at baseline. Despite high levels of pain, ZB quickly acquired reclined and upright relaxed behavior, though upright relaxation proved more challenging. Both reclined and upright relaxation was maintained at the three-month follow-up assessment.

Pain anxiety scores (PASS) for each of four sub-scales are shown in Figure 6.2. In baseline, three scales were relatively stable while the Physiological scale showed a marked increase. All scales showed a steady decline over the

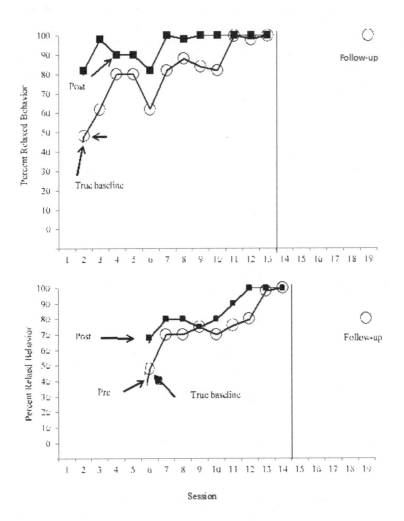

Figure 6.1 Pre-post percent relaxed behavior in the reclined and upright positions.

Based on Lundervold, D.A., Talley, C., & Buermann, M. (2006). Effect of behavioral activation treatment on Fibromyalgia related pain anxiety cognition. *International Journal of Behavioral Consultation and Therapy, 2*(1), 73–84.

course of the BAT-P intervention, which included reclined and upright BRT, and remained at low levels at follow-up.

Similarly, Pain Interference ratings (PIR) showed a decrease over the course of the BAT-P intervention (Figure 6.3). Some spikes occurred, particularly when ZB experienced a migraine shortly after the start of training. But the overall trend was downward, with good maintenance at follow-up.

Figure 6.4 displays self-reported depression scores based on the GDS-15. ZB was severely depressed during baseline assessment. As she gained skills in increasing relaxation and accessing valued events and activities, along with decreasing pain, her depression remitted. Her score was well below the clinical cut-off at follow-up. A medication index (MI) score was calculated using baseline, end-of-treatment and follow-up reports of medication usage. MI scores showed a slight decline from baseline to end of treatment. However, comparison of MI scores for follow-up was not possible due to a change in medication.

FIBROMYALGIA AND CHRONIC BACK PAIN. Janet, a 46-year-old woman, married and employed, had an extensive history of chronic pain including

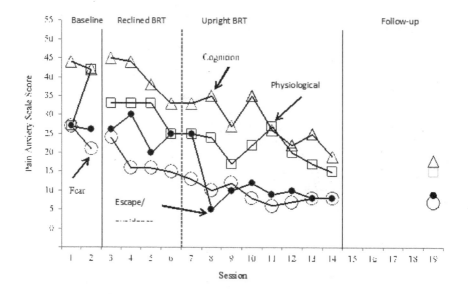

Figure 6.2 Pain Anxiety Cognition Symptom Scale (PASS) scores across conditions.
Based on Lundervold, D.A., Talley, C., & Buermann, M. (2006). Effect of behavioral activation treatment on fibromyalgia-related pain anxiety cognition. International Journal of Behavioral Consultation and Therapy, 2(1), 73–84.

PAIN AND ANXIETY DISORDERS • 161

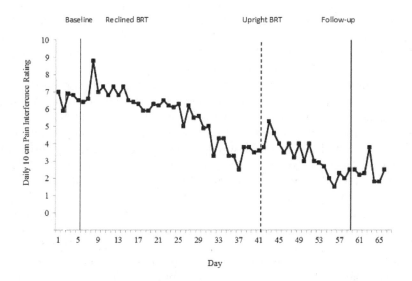

Figure 6.3 Daily pain interference rating (PIR) across conditions.
Lundervold, D.A., Talley, C., & Buermann, M. (2006). Effect of behavioral activation treatment on fibromyalgia-related pain anxiety cognition. *International Journal of Behavioral Consultation and Therapy,* 2(1), 73–84.

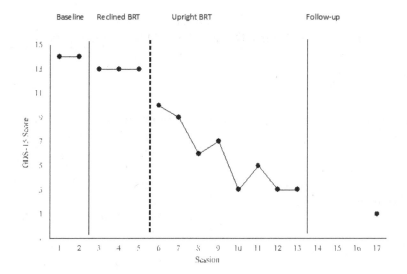

Figure 6.4 Geriatric Depression Scale-15 (GDS-15) across conditions.
Lundervold, D.A., Talley, C., & Buermann, M. (2006). Effect of behavioral activation treatment on fibromyalgia-related pain anxiety cognition. *International Journal of Behavioral Consultation and Therapy,* 2(1), 73–84.

FM, lower and upper back, migraine headache, and abdominal pain. She frequently used anxiolytics, antidepressant, analgesic and narcotic pain medications. Janet had undergone surgery to fuse her cervical vertebrae. Her low-back pain was related to bulging disks secondary to congenital degeneration of the spine and vertebrae. (See Table 6.1).

Assessment, as with ZB, included self-report scales of pain interference (PIR), depression (GDS-15), pain anxiety (PASS), and medication usage. Baseline measurements of relaxed behavior (BRS) for both Reclined and Upright positions were collected across four initial evaluation sessions. Janet then reported that she was scheduled for more back surgery, resulting in a six-week hiatus while she recovered. Two more baseline sessions were conducted in which Reclined and Upright BRS measures were taken.

Treatment was similar to that described for ZB, in which the BAT-P procedures were carried out in the context of BRT in both Reclined and Upright positions. The relaxed behaviors were taught in two sets of five behaviors each, for both Reclined and Upright BRT, in a multiple-baseline-across-behavior-sets design. This allowed one to see if training on Set 1 had any influence (e.g., enhancement or inhibition) on training Set 2. Set 1 was comprised of Body, Head, Shoulders, Hands, and Feet. Set 2 included Breathing, Quiet, Eyes, Mouth and Throat. Reclined BRT was taught first, with several probe assessments in the Upright position. Then Upright BRT was taught.

Table 6.1
Medical Conditions, Duration, and Medication Regimen

Medical Condition	Duration	Medication
Congenital degenerative disks	15 years	Ultram: 50 mg every six hours Zanaflex: 4 mg six hours Ativan: 10 mg nightly PRN
Fibromyalgia	22 years	Hydrocodone: 5/500 mg every six hours Trazadone: 50 mg once a day
Migraine headache	20 years	
Irritable Bowel Syndrome	10 years	

Based on Lundervold, D. A., Talley, C., & Buermann, M. (2008). Effect of behavioral treatment on chronic fibrymyalia pain: Replication and extension. *International Journal of Behavioral Consultation and Therapy,* 4(2), 146–157.

Janet's BRS scores are shown in Figure 6.5. The pre-surgery baseline is designated A1 and post-surgery is A2. After the baseline measurements, reclined BRT was implemented, concurrent with shaping participation in valued behavioral activities and the other BAT-P components as described in the previous case of ZB. After the reclined behaviors were acquired, upright

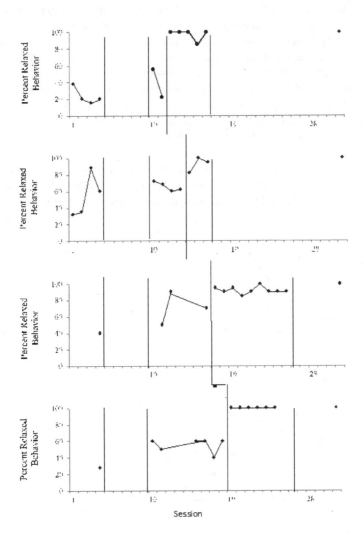

Figure 6.5 Percent relaxed behavior across behavior sets and reclined and upright positions.
Based on Lundervold, D.A., Talley, C., & Buermann, M. (2008). Effect of behavioral activation treatment on chronic fibromyalgia pain: Replication and extension. *International Journal of Behavioral Consultation and Therapy*, 4(2), 146–157.

relaxed postures were taught and combined with the remaining BAT-P components.

Baseline assessment of reclined and upright relaxed behavior indicated variable performance in both positions, with behavior sets in the reclined and upright position resulting in relatively poor BRS scores (see Figure 6.5). Performance in in the A2 condition, following surgery, was generally lower than A1. Four sets of relaxed behaviors—two reclined and two upright—were taught to Janet. While teaching Reclined Set 1, baseline assessment of Reclined Set 2, and Upright Set 1 and 2 remained in baseline. Once stability in performance for Reclined Set 1 was observed, instruction of Reclined Set 2 commenced, and so on for Upright Set 1 and 2. BAT-P components were implemented concurrent with instruction of Reclined Behavior Set 1 and were continuously implemented as more relaxed behaviors were acquired. Homework was given each session in the manner described for ZB.

Figure 6.6 displays the relative effects of reclined and upright BRT on pain-anxiety in the context of the BAT-P intervention. PASS scores were high during the A1 condition, with cognitive and physiological anxiety higher than escape/avoidance and fear, though scores on all four dimensions

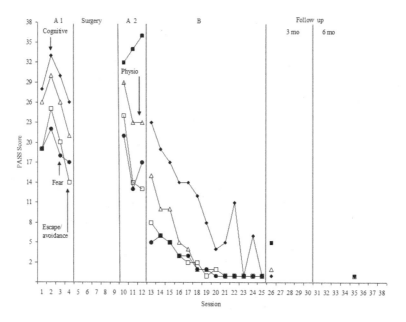

Figure 6.6. PASS scores during baseline (A1, A2), reclined and upright BRT in the context of BAT-P (B) and at a six-month follow up.

Based on Lundervold, D.A., Talley, C., & Buermann, M. (2008). Effect of behavioral activation treatment on chronic fibromyalgia pain: Replication and extension. *International Journal of Behavioral Consultation and Therapy*, 4(2), 146–157.

declined with further assessment. PASS scores remained relatively stable after surgery, though physiological anxiety increased to its highest level. An immediate effect of reclined BRT was observed on each of the four PASS sub-scale scores following the first BRT Session. They continued to decline with further training. With the initiation of Upright BRT, PASS scores appeared to decrease in variability, except for physiological anxiety, which was the trailing indicator of distress. While more variable than the other three PASS scores, physiological anxiety eventually reached zero levels. Zero levels of pain anxiety were observed at the six-month follow-up as well.

Janet suffered extreme pain interference, with the majority of her baseline PIR scores above 7.5, as shown in Figure 6.7. Her post-surgery PIR scores were equally high. Reclined BRT resulted in an immediate decline in her PIR scores, followed by variable increases and decreases. In the latter part of the Reclined BRT phase, PIR scores steadily declined. With the implementation of Upright BRT, PIR scores stabilized and ranged from .5 cm to 2.75 cm. One spike in pain interference occurred in the UBRT-BAT-P condition, but rating quickly returned to their previous low level. PIR scores at the six-month follow-up were lower than at the end of BAT-P.

With BRT based BAT-P, Janet was able to reduce her medication usage from the A1 baseline MI score of 39.71, indicating a high usage of medications. The MI score (64.57) for the A2, the post-surgery baseline, was substantially higher. Janet's end-of-treatment MI score based on the last week of

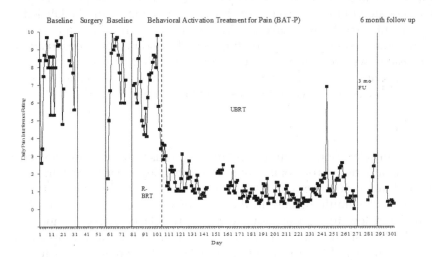

Figure 6.7 Daily pain inference rating during reclined and upright BRT in the context of BAT-P.
Based on Lundervold, D.A., Talley, C., & Buermann, M. (2008). Effect of behavioral activation treatment on chronic fibromyalgia pain: Replication and extension. *International Journal of Behavioral Consultation and Therapy*, 4(2), 146–157.

intervention, was 23.62. Medication usage at six-month follow up was markedly reduced (13.00).

Summary

Pain is a complex phenomenon that often brings on anxiety or depression when medication or other efforts to alleviate it are not successful. Pain is multi-modal, with elements in the motor (e.g., muscle tension), visceral (e.g., vascular derangement in migraine), verbal (e.g., "This is killing me!"), and observational (e.g., focus of attention) realms. Sometimes relaxation itself may provide a sufficient antidote, but often additional programmatic efforts (like the BAT-P) are needed to encourage the participant to utilize relaxation and other skills to engage a more reinforcing environment. As noted in so many other instances, BRT is an effective and efficient method to teach relaxation skills. And the BRS and other measures provide feedback to both the therapist and the participant on the progress they are making.

ANXIETY DISORDERS

As described in Chapter 1, anxiety is a pervasive and costly affliction. It may vary from specific phobias of particular objects or situations to generalized feelings of dread or overwhelming occurrences of panic. Anxiety is also related to the occurrence of chronic illness and would be labeled an adjustment disorder with anxiety. As presented in Chapter 2, anxiety is a multimodal response, across motor, verbal, visceral, and observational dimensions, with relaxation providing functional alternatives in each dimension. Relaxation training, in various guises, has a long history in the treatment of anxiety. This section focuses on the use of BRT.

Phobia

The use of relaxation to counteract anxious arousal in response to specific stimulus situations is one of the founding principles of behavior therapy.[34,35] The technique of *systematic desensitization* involves presenting a series of fear-evoking stimuli, usually in the form of verbal description, in a hierarchy from low to high arousal, to a deeply relaxed person. Thousands of published studies attest to the efficacy of this procedure. Most of this research employs PMR to teach relaxation, but BRT would appear to be at least equally effective.

FEAR OF CROSSING BRIDGES IN AN ADULT MAN. Helfer[36] was one of the first to use BRT in a standard systematic desensitization.[34] Mr. A, age 30, employed and married with two children, was referred by his physician for phobic anxiety. In a clinical interview, Mr. A reported a fear of crossing bridges since childhood, but could recall no precipitating event. The Fear Survey Schedule (FSS)[37] was administered, on which Mr. A reported fear of heights and of blood/injury. The bridge phobia interfered with his social and family life because he avoided automobile trips that required crossing bridges. In instances where it was absolutely necessary, his wife or a friend drove while he closed his eyes and experienced trembling, sweating, difficulty concentrating, and embarrassment. Highway overpasses in the course of driving to work were not a problem. Mr. A was given a rationale for systematic desensitization emphasizing the incompatibility between relaxation and anxiety.

The first two sessions were devoted to gathering information, and after each Mr. A was asked to relax as he normally did, providing baseline BRS data. The next ten sessions involved fear-hierarchy construction and BRT. Training duration was about 20 minutes. Although he learned the relaxed behaviors quickly, Mr. A reported great discomfort in being observed and "evaluated." After three sessions, only positive, rather than corrective feedback was provided.

A 19-item stimulus hierarchy was constructed, involving dimensions of people present in the car, person driving, particular bridges, time before a trip, proximity to or location on a bridge, and day or night. Mr. A rated each item on a 100-point Subjective Unit of Distress Scale (SUD)[34] and items were arranged to produce a progression from low- to high-fear items. In addition, three high-intensity items (90 to 100 SUD) were employed as probe stimuli, inserted at various points throughout the desensitization program to determine his response to scenes presented out of sequence.

During the desensitization phase, Mr. A relaxed for 10 minutes followed by about 15 minutes of scene presentation. He was asked to vividly imagine a scene read by the therapist, to signal by raising his index finger when he had a clear image of the scene, and to use the same signal if he became anxious while imagining it. Each item was presented three times for successive durations of 15, 30, and 45 seconds, with approximately 30 to 60 seconds between presentations. If he exhibited additional unrelaxed behavior while imagining a scene, then the therapist provided appropriate relaxation instructions before presenting the next item. Each session began with the last scene successfully imagined in the previous session. In the middle of the third, fifth, and seventh desensitization sessions (Sessions 15, 17, and 19), probe items were presented for 45 seconds.

Desensitization proceeded smoothly for Mr. A. He never signaled discomfort for an item, even when the high-intensity probes were presented. After completion of the hierarchy, the therapist took two trips with Mr. A, driving over large bridges that crossed the Mississippi River, each about 60 miles round-trip. On both occasions, Mr. A displayed and reported no anxiety. He was smiling and relaxed, and commented on how easy it felt.

Figure 6.8 shows BRS scores for Mr. A during Baseline (A), BRT (B), and Desensitization (C) phases. The BRS was scored during training and scene presentation. Note that these are measures of *un*relaxed behavior, so decreasing values indicate better relaxation. Rapid improvement occurred over the first three training sessions, even though Mr. A reported subjective discomfort, as shown in Figure 6.9. The change to the positive-feedback only procedure (on Session 6) resulted in slight increases in unrelaxed behaviors but improvements in self-report. Desensitization commenced after four BRT sessions in which self-report was 3 ("Feeling more relaxed than usual") or better.

Unrelaxed behavior remained low during desensitization, but showed a marked increase when one probe item was presented in Session 17, suggesting some arousal. However, Mr. A remained relaxed with the other probe items on Sessions 15 and 19. And his self-report remained low during all probe presentations.

Three months later, a follow-up was conducted. His score on the FSS showed a marked decrease on items related to crossing bridges as well as

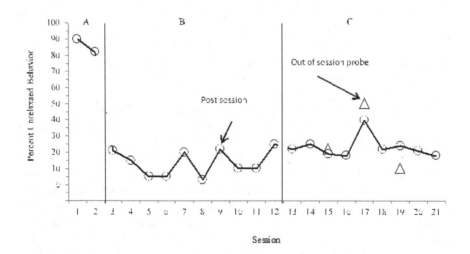

Figure 6.8 Percentage of unrelaxed behaviors across conditions.

Based on Helfer, S. L. (1984). *Systematic desensitization with behavioral relaxation training: Assessment of cognitive, physiological, and behavioral response systems.* Unpublished master's thesis, Southern Illinois University at Carbondale.

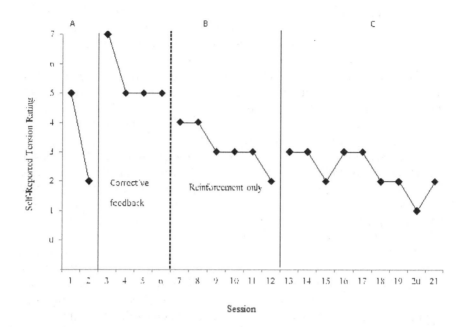

Figure 6.9. Self-reported discomfort across conditions.

Based on Helfer, S. L. (1984). *Systematic desensitization with behavioral relaxation training: Assessment of cognitive, physiological, and behavioral response systems.* Unpublished master's thesis, Southern Illinois University at Carbondale.

to blood/injury, with no change on heights. He reported he'd made several bridge crossings, as either driver or passenger, with no negative feelings, and expressed great satisfaction with expanded family and social activities this new freedom allowed.

FEAR OF FLYING IN AN OLDER MAN WITH NEUROCOGNITIVE IMPAIRMENT. Acute and chronic medical conditions are related to anxiety across the lifespan.[38-40] Twenty-five percent of older adults with minor neurocognitive impairment (M-NCI) report anxious arousal.[41-43] Despite the high percentage of older adults with M-NCI who suffer distress, there is a dearth of literature describing treatment of M-NCI and anxiety generally, and no reports describing treatment of M-NCI and specific phobia.

Chuck[44] was 69 years old and had 16 years of education. Based on a battery of norm-referenced cognitive assessments, he was diagnosed with minor neurocognitive impairment, probable Alzheimer's disease, with behavioral disturbance. He had a history of a specific phobia related to airplane travel but reported that he had been able to manage it using distraction procedures.

During his last holiday, however, he had significant difficulty during a trip, including a mild altercation with the flight attendant due to anxiety while seated on the plane. He reported serious fear about an upcoming airline trip in approximately three weeks.

Chuck had never received counseling or therapy for his fear and had refused anxiolytic medication because of concerns about substance dependence and a general aversion to medication. However, he did agree to and was stabilized on 10 mg of Donepezil for cognitive impairment. Behavioral treatment was provided in an integrated geriatric primary care setting.

The first session was devoted to clarifying the fear-related situations and development of a preliminary fear hierarchy. Brief imaginal exposure and relaxation was explained to Chuck and his approval was obtained. During the second session, refinement of the fear hierarchy and SUD ratings for each scene was completed. Baseline reclined relaxed behavior was assessed using the BRS for a two-minute direct observation period.

Sessions were conducted twice a week. Two 20-minute sessions of reclined BRT were conducted. Chuck was instructed to practice relaxation on his own twice per day and make daily pre-post ratings of relaxation, which were then reviewed at the next session. Three sessions of BRT and brief imaginal exposure (BIE) were then conducted. Each exposure trial was two minutes in duration, with each scene presented three to four times. Each session began with two minutes of reclined BRT proficiency training, followed by BIE. Chuck was instructed to continue to relax and to imagine as clearly as possible the situation described by the therapist. A script for each scene, derived from the fear hierarchy, was used to ensure consistency in exposure content. At the end of each scene, Chuck was asked to report his SUD rating. Immediately following the rating, he was instructed to "erase that scene from your mind" and to continue to relax. Progression to the next scene occurred contingent on a reduction in the SUD rating. Immediately prior to presenting the next scene in the hierarchy, a two-minute direct observation of relaxed behavior was conducted. During the final two sessions, upright relaxed behaviors were demonstrated, followed by imitation with corrective feedback and praise. Chuck was encouraged to use upright relaxed postures while seated in the airplane. A written description of each of the upright relaxed behaviors was provided as a prompt.

Despite his cognitive impairment, Chuck easily acquired the relaxed behaviors which were maintained at each post-BEI observation (see Figure 6.10). The standard BRT acquisition criterion of 80 percent was achieved and maintained on 66 percent of the post-BIE observations of relaxed behavior. Figure 6.11 displays pre-post SUD ratings related to each feared situation. Baseline (Pre-BIE) SUD ratings increased in intensity, which formed the

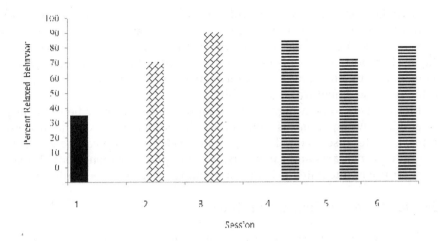

Figure 6.10 Percent relaxed behavior during baseline and reclined BRT.
Lundervold, D.A. & Holt, P.S. (2011). *Brief imaginal exposure for specific phobia with an older adult with mild cognitive impairment (MCI) with amnesia.* Anxiety and Depression Association of America, San Jose, CA.

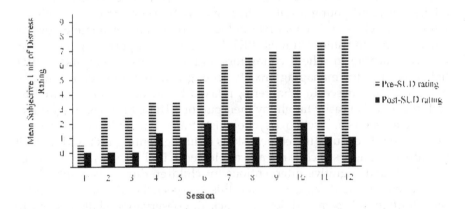

Figure 6.11 Mean subject unit of distress (SUD) rating at baseline and after brief imaginal exposure (BIE) with reclined BRT.
Lundervold, D.A. & Holt, P.S. (2011). *Brief imaginal exposure for specific phobia with an older adult with mild cognitive impairment (MCI) with amnesia.* Anxiety and Depression Association of America, San Jose, CA.

basis for the hierarchy. Low (Post-BIE) SUD ratings were observed following training, when Chuck imagined the scenes while relaxed.

Four days after the last BIE session, Chuck completed a cross-country flight. He reported one episode of distress, with a SUD rating of 1, which he managed by engaging in upright relaxation. Unfortunately, systematic follow-up assessment was not possible.

BRT appears to be a highly effective procedure that may benefit many older adults with phobia, as well as for older adults with NCI and anxious arousal.[41-43] Because reclined and upright relaxed posture can be so easily taught to participants and caregivers, it is an optimal evidence-based treatment for use in integrated primary care settings serving older adults.[45]

BRT for Anxiety in Educational Settings

The prevalence of anxiety disorders among those 13 to 18 years of age is reported to be over 30 percent[2], with over eight percent severely impaired and females at greater risk. A significant number of children, adolescents, and young adults also suffer from test anxiety.[46,47] Professionals in educational settings have a great opportunity to effect change among children, adolescents, and young adults suffering anxiety. With increasing calls for school counselors and school psychologists to use and evaluate evidence-based counseling interventions, BRT becomes an important intervention readily available to school counselors and school psychologists.[48-50] BRT holds promise for managing anxiety among children and adolescents,[51,52] because, as discussed in Chapter 5, relaxed behavior can be acquired by children and also easily taught by their parents. These findings suggest that school counselors and school psychologists trained in evidence-based practices can easily acquire the clinical skills of implementing BRT and using it to address the needs of children and adolescents. BRT also has an advantage over PMR and cognitive interventions for children due to its emphasis on overt behavior. As discussed earlier, this is especially advantageous given that children and some adolescents lack the observation skills needed to notice covert behavior, such as anxious self-talk. While relaxation is a component in evidence-based cognitive behavior therapy for children and adolescents with anxiety, relaxation skills acquired through BRT are easier to learn and don't require the tense-relax exercises of PMR that children may find difficult to perform.

ANXIETY IN HIGH SCHOOL STUDENTS. Rashid and Parish[53] compared the effects of upright BRT, PMR, and a no-treatment control group in a between-groups experimental design with high school students. Indirect measures of

State and Trait Anxiety were obtained using Speilberger's[54] State-Trait Inventory. Eighteen students were assigned to the BRT condition; twenty to PMR; and seventeen to no-treatment control. Group relaxation training was conducted using a video modeling the procedures and instruction with a male and female alternating as trainer and participant. Students were then asked to imitate the relaxed behaviors or perform the tense-release exercises, depending on group assignment. Four twenty-minute training sessions over a two-week period were conducted. Assessment occurred one day after the last training session. No assessment of relaxed behavior or self-reported tension, pre- or post-training sessions was obtained. Students were not instructed to practice relaxation between sessions.

A 3x2 analysis of variance of anxiety scores indicated a significant main effect of treatment, and no effect of gender or gender x treatment interaction for State Anxiety. Both BRT and PMR resulted in lower State Anxiety scores compared to controls. Post hoc results indicated no significant difference between BRT and PMR. No significant effect was observed for Trait Anxiety. Rashid and Parish recommended BRT as the preferred relaxation procedure for school counselors to use because of its efficiency and effectiveness.

TEST ANXIETY IN UNDERGRADUATE STUDENTS. Test anxiety has been shown to impair academic performance. According to Chapell et al.,[55] high-test-anxious undergraduate students are likely to score 33 percent lower than their non-test-anxious counterparts. Tatum, Lundervold and Ament[56] examined the effect of abbreviated upright BRT with a sample of undergraduate students who reported test anxiety.

Twenty self-referred undergraduate female students took part, ten each in treatment and control groups. The participants ranged in age from eighteen to forty years of age. Measures of subjective distress (SUD ratings), using a 10-point scale, and test anxiety, using the Abbreviated Test Anxiety Scale (ATAS), were obtained. The ATAS was a slightly modified version of the Abbreviated Math Test Anxiety Scale.[57] It focused on anxious feelings during exams and quizzes with scores ranging from 9 to 45.

At Time 1, all participants completed the ATAS. For the experimental group, two 30-minute group sessions of upright BRT were conducted in a classroom, using standard student desks. Acquisition of the ten behaviors occurred in the first session. Following a short break, the next 30 minutes was used for proficiency training. Contingent praise and feedback were provided for relaxed behaviors. No BRS scores or self-reports of tension were obtained. Those in the BRT condition were encouraged to practice and use relaxation prior to and during quizzes or exams they may have in the coming week. No treatment was provided for the control group.

Over the ensuing week, all participants were asked to record a SUD rating immediately prior to each quiz or exam while seated in the classroom. At Time 2, one week later, the ATAS was once again completed by everyone and SUD ratings were collected. Participants in the no-treatment control condition completed the ATAS at T1, recorded SUD ratings between sessions and again completed the ATAS at T2. No follow-up assessment was possible due to the end of the academic semester.

SUD ratings for exams/quizzes ranged from one to four in the period between T1 and T2. Independent *t*-tests for of ATAS scores for the BRT and no-treatment control group were nonsignificant ($p = <.10$). Results of the independent *t*-test comparing T2 SUD and ATAS scores of the experiment and control group were significant with lower scores obtained for the BRT group (See Figure 6.12). The BRT group also had significantly lower SUD rating. (See Figure 6.13).

Tatum et al. demonstrated that upright relaxed postures could be taught quickly using standard materials found in a university classroom in a group context without the need for high technology such as video recordings. The strength of the research lies in use of a no-treatment control group and repeated measurement using *in situ* distress ratings and validated self-report measures. With further training and practice of BRT, it would be expected that greater improvement in SUD ratings and ATAS scores would be observed.

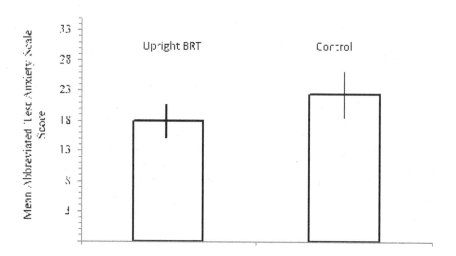

Figure 6.12 Mean Abbreviated Test Anxiety Scale score and standard deviation for the experimental and control group.

Based on Tatum, T., Lundervold, D.A., Ament, P.A. (2006). Abbreviated Upright Behavioral Relaxation Training for test anxiety among college students: Initial results. *International Journal of Behavioral Consultation and Therapy*, 2(4), 475–479.

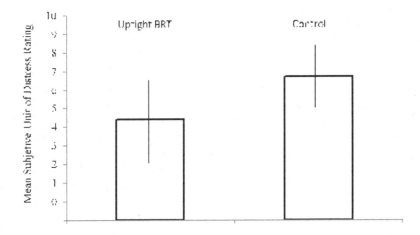

Figure 6.13 Mean subjective unit of distress rating and standard deviation for the experimental and control groups.
Based on Tatum, T., Lundervold, D.A., Ament, P.A. (2006). Abbreviated Upright Behavioral Relaxation Training for test anxiety among college students: Initial results. *International Journal of Behavioral Consultation and Therapy*, 2(4), 475–479.

Anxiety Related to Movement Disorders

Movement disorders are neurological conditions that affect the speed, fluency and accuracy of movement. The motor action may be hyper- or hypokinetic, ballistic, sustained, or repetitive. Despite movement disorders tending to be heritable conditions, it is well know that the magnitude of functional disability is exacerbated by environmental events such as stress, task demands, emotional arousal, and observation by others.[58-60] Because the disordered movement is publicly observable, individuals with a movement disorder can easily become stigmatized. Over the past 20 years, there has been a growing awareness of the non-motor symptoms of movement disorders such as anxiety and depression and their relation to impaired movement.[61-64] The prevalence of anxiety disorders among movement disorder participants is high and varies depending on the specific type of anxiety. For example, Wenzel, Schnider, Wimmer et al.[65] reported that approximately 30 percent of participants with dystonia met diagnostic criteria for one or more anxiety disorders. Social anxiety is also pervasive among participants with essential tremor and ranges from 30 to 33 percent among non-clinic samples.[66, 67]

As relaxation has been shown to be an evidenced-based treatment for anxiety disorders among individuals without disordered movement, it would appear that individuals with movement disorders and anxiety would also benefit. Due to the impaired neurological system regulating the voluntary control of the muscles, the use of progressive relaxation procedures would be contraindicated. Because BRT does not require the tense-release actions of PMR, it is ideally suited for use with participants with movement disorders and anxiety.

PARKINSON'S DISEASE (PD). Parkinson's disease (PD) is a progressive degenerative movement disorder with both motor and non-motor symptoms, with peak onset occurring between the ages of 60 and 69. Research indicates that a number of behavioral and environmental factors are predictive of anxiety and depression among participants with PD, including limited problem-focused coping skills and decreased social support (social reinforcement for healthy behavior).[68] While awareness of the non-motor symptoms of PD has increased, anxiety remains under-recognized and under-treated.[69,70] Fortunately, the benefits of relaxation-based interventions for non-motor symptoms of PD is increasing.[71-75]

PD, dyskinesia, and anxiety: Beth.
Beth[75] was a 57-year-old woman who, 18 months prior, had undergone a deep brain stimulation implant (DBS) of her sub-thalamic nucleus to decrease motor impairment from PD. However, surgery had little effect on her dyskinesia, which consisted of involuntary movements in her right lower leg. Dyskinesia was evoked by stressful social situations and driving in heavy traffic. Beth had no previous history of anxiety, and psychological assessment prior to DBS surgery indicated no psychopathology. She was stabilized on anti-Parkinson and anxiolytic medication for six months prior to referral. Table 6.2 describes her clinical status using the United Parkinson's Disease Rating Scale[76] conducted prior to DBS surgery. Post-DBS UPDRS assessment revealed significant functional improvement and mild to minimal dyskinesia.

Because Beth resided four hours away from the point of service, and her time in the city was spent seeing multiple health care providers, brief, intensive behavioral intervention was provided. Five visits occurred, each approximately 45 minutes in duration, two to four weeks apart. A follow-up visit was scheduled six weeks after the fifth session.

Beth was first completed the Geriatric Depression Scale-Long Form (GDS-LF),[77] and the Clinical Anxiety Scale (CAS).[78] She then she took part in a behavioral interview which served as a function-based assessment to pinpoint intervention goals, target behaviors, and current maintaining antecedent and consequent conditions related to anxiety and dyskinesia.

Functional-based assessment indicated that her anxiety was elicited by dyskinesia occurring in stressful situations. It appeared that PD functioned as a biological setting event[79] that modulated the strength of her reflexive leg movement (unconditioned response) to environmental stressors (uncondi-

Table 6.2
UPDRS scores with and without DBS stimulation and medication regimen.

Medication	Years since diagnosis	Mentation	UPDRS[1] ADL On[2] / Off	UPDRS[1] Motor On / Off	PD Stage[3]
MVIqd Prevacid 15mg Colace 1qd Amantadine 100 mg tid Artane 2 mg tid Lexapro 10 mg qid Sinemet 25/100 ½, 5x/day Ambien 5 mg qhs prn Fosamax 1 q week	11 years 2 months	Mild confusion Intermittent depression	6 7	14 19	H/Y 3/4

[1] UPDRS with stimulation at the time of behavior therapy
[2] UPDRS assessment conducted stimulation on/off
[3] Hoehn & Yahr (1967) disease severity staging

Based on Lundervold, D.A., Pahwa, R. Lyons, K.E. (2013). Behavioral Relaxation Training for Parkinson's Disease related dyskinesia and comorbid social anxiety. *International Journal of Behavioral Consultation and Therapy*, 7(4), 1–5.

tioned stimulus: car traffic). Under these conditions, she became very anxious, and soon the car traffic would elicit anxiety prior to dyskinesia. Beth had started to avoid social situations and drive less frequently, and became increasingly anxious when she had to drive in the city.

Beth was instructed in Upright BRT immediately following the behavioral interview. The Upright position was employed because she reported that both anxiety and dyskinesia occurred when she was seated, especially while driving. A rationale for self-recording distress was provided and she was taught how to make SUD ratings using a 10-point scale. She was encouraged to practice relaxation at least once a day and to use it in anxiety-provoking situations or as soon as she noticed dyskinesia occurring. She was instructed to continue relaxing until her distress declined or the dyskinesia lessened, at which point she recorded pre-post relaxation SUD ratings. Recording forms were mailed or hand delivered depending on the date of the next visit.

At the start of each subsequent session, Beth's homework was reviewed and any problems discussed. This was followed by approximately twenty minutes of Upright BRT to reinforce her relaxation skills.

At baseline assessment, Beth's score on the GDS-LF was below the clinical cut-off and declined further over the course of BRT. Her baseline CAS score (35) indicated mild anxiety and declined to below the clinical cut-off score by the end of BRT (11), with low reported levels of anxiety (CAS 8) maintained at the six-week follow-up. Beth rapidly acquired the Upright relaxed behaviors and improved with each booster session. She was also successful in managing her anxiety *in vivo* by using upright relaxation. Figure 6.14 shows weekly averages of her SUD scores when facing a provoking situation and after relaxing to deal with it. Beth also reported that BRT was highly acceptable to her as an intervention for the anxiety and dyskinesia.[80]

PD, dyskinesia, and anxiety: Ralph.
Ralph,[81] age 67, wrestled with the challenges of early onset PD that had afflicted him since age 49 and was becoming worse. His PD was complicated by anxiety that began to occur thirteen years earlier. Because of his long history of dopaminergic medication, it had begun to lose its effectiveness in controlling the PD symptoms, resulting in dyskinesia.[82] His most recent Unified Parkinson's Disease Rating Scale (UPDRS) evaluation indicated that he suffered from mild confusion, forgetfulness, and motor impairment. He had

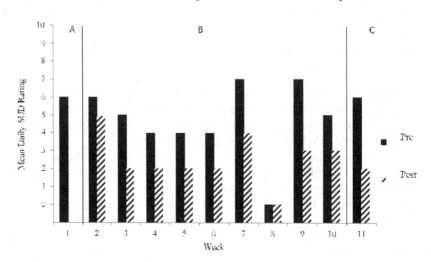

Figure 6.14 Mean pre-post relaxation SUD ratings in baseline (A), in situ with BRT (B), and follow-up (C).

Based on Lundervold, D.A., Pahwa, R. Lyons, K.E. (2013). Behavioral Relaxation Training for Parkinson's Disease related dyskinesia and comorbid social anxiety. *International Journal of Behavioral Consultation and Therapy*, 7(4), 1–5.

severe upper extremity dyskinesia and suffered bouts of anxiety. Ralph had been a candidate for DBS surgery, but it was postponed due to his anxiety and poor performance on neuropsychological tests. An experimental brain surgery procedure was available to him if he could manage his anxiety more effectively and test results were more favorable. Testing and surgery were scheduled six weeks from the time he sought treatment. He reported that this limited time added to his anxiety.

Twice-weekly sessions were conducted up until two days prior to assessment for surgery. Ralph was provided with a biobehavioral conceptualization of anxiety followed by a rationale for multi-method behavioral assessment. Measures of anxiety (CAS) and depression (GDS) were completed at the start of each session. It was decided to use Upright BRT because Ralph had difficulty rising from a recliner. Following a five-minute adaptation period, a five-minute observation of Upright BRS was conducted. Finally, Ralph was taught to use the 10-point SUD rating scale and instructed to make ratings four times daily (breakfast, lunch, supper, bedtime), and episodically if an upsetting event occurred.

Two sessions of Upright BRT were conducted. The relaxed behaviors were taught in two sets of five behaviors each (Set 1: Body, Head, Shoulders, Hands, and Feet; Set 2: Breathing, Quiet, Eyes, Mouth and Throat). Each BRT session lasted approximately 20 minutes and was followed by the post-training observation in which both behavior sets were scored concurrently. After the observation, Ralph was asked how he felt, what he noticed while relaxing, and what behavior was most difficult for him to relax. Feedback and praise were provided contingent on his report. At the end of each session, Ralph was instructed to practice Upright BRT once per day for 15 minutes and encouraged to relax whenever he felt anxious. His wife was asked to observe and record his relaxation using the Caregiver Relaxation Checklist (Appendix J). This entailed observing him for two minutes while he relaxed and scoring his behavior using the checklist.

To make further progress and minimize the disruptive effects of Ralph's within-session dyskinesia, BRT was combined with pleasant images that had been derived from discussion. Ralph first relaxed for five minutes, as he had been taught. Then guided imagery was alternated with praise and feedback every 60 seconds.

The last two sessions were devoted to BRT and coping within the context of the neuropsychological examination. As before, Ralph was asked to relax on his own for five minutes, with contingent praise and feedback provided. This was followed by BRT plus imaginal exposure to the neuropsychological test situation. Ralph was instructed to imagine a sequence of situations leading up to being at the exam table on the day of the testing and taking the various tests. Each situation was described to Ralph while he relaxed. He was also instructed to "relax away the anxiety" whenever he began to feel an increase in tension and anxiety. A post-training observation of relaxed behavior occurred after each BRT + Coping session. Again, Ralph was encouraged to practice and use the relaxation at home and during the testing.

Ralph's severe dyskinesia prevented his attaining the standard BRT criterion of 80 percent relaxed. As seen in Figure 6.15, relaxed behaviors in Set

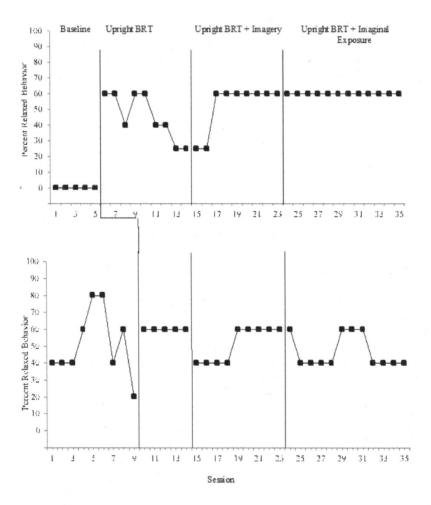

Figure 6.15 Percent relaxed behavior across upright relaxed behavior sets.

Based on Lundervold, D. A., Pahwa, R. Lyons, K. E. (2009). Effect of Behavioral Relaxation training on comorbid general anxiety disorder and Parkinson's disease. *Clinical Gerontologist, 32*, 104–117.

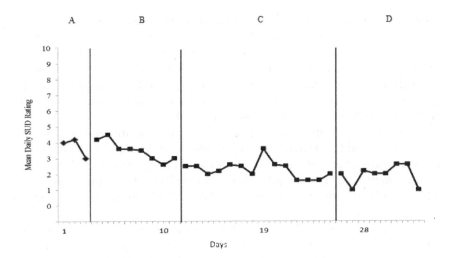

Figure 6.16 Mean daily SUD rating during baseline (A), Upright BRT (B), Upright BRT + imagery (C), and Upright BRT + imaginal exposure (D).

Based on Lundervold, D. A., Pahwa, R. Lyons, K. E. (2009). Effect of Behavioral Relaxation training on comorbid general anxiety disorder and Parkinson's disease. *Clinical Gerontologist, 32*, 104–117.

1 increased from zero to 60 percent, and became more stable in the Imagery and Coping phases. Behaviors in Set 2 occurred at a higher frequency in Baseline and never exceeded 60 percent relaxed.

Mean daily SUD ratings, Figure 6.16, showed a steady decline across phases. *Baseline-corrected TAU (B-TAU)* is a means of analyzing changes in performance across phases in single-subject designs while controlling for a trend in the data.[83,84] Analysis of SUD ratings indicated a statistically significant difference between A (Baseline) and B (UBRT) [$B\text{-}TAU = .67, p = .02$], and between B and C (UBRT + Imagery) [$B\text{-}TAU = .60, p = .001$]. No difference was found between phases C and D (UBRT + Coping).

An independent assessor rated Ralph's level of anxiety during the neuropsychological testing and reported that his anxiety was no greater than other participants in that situation. That Ralph was able to manage his anxiety during testing provided social validity data to support the BRT treatment package used.

Essential Tremor (ET)

ET and anxiety: Wanda.

Wanda, a 62-year-old woman with ET, was very concerned that she was developing PD, for which she had a family history. She had been diagnosed with voice, hand, and head tremor for about four years, and reported that they had recently gotten worse. She also complained of feeling paralyzed for several seconds after awaking from sleep, provoking a feeling of dread. According to the most recent neurological evaluation, Wanda had ET and mild functional disability. Xanax was prescribed by her neurologist but she discontinued it and refused further anxiolytic medication. No medication for tremor was prescribed. Wanda resided six hours away from the point of contact so visits were initially scheduled monthly.

The behavioral interview on her initial visit identified: (a) behavioral sequelae related to ET; (b) degree of emotional distress; (c) antecedents and consequences of anxiety and dysphoria; and (d) treatment goals and intervention methods. She was administered the Clinical Anxiety Scale (CAS = 32) and the Geriatric Depression Scale (GDS-15 = 7), indicating mild anxiety and depression.

Wanda was educated on the differences between PD and ET and how stress affected ET. Multiple stressors that affected her functioning were identified, including her fear of PD, her husband's health problems, her children's marital problems, interacting with others in public, and performing her job as a teacher. A biobehavioral conceptualization of ET was presented along with a rationale and outcome expectation for the effects of BRT.

Also on the initial visit, Upright BRT was conducted, beginning with a five-minute baseline, in which Wanda was instructed simply to relax in a straight back chair as she normally would. Next, for approximately twenty minutes, instruction in the ten relaxed behaviors was provided. Each behavior was taught to Wanda as described in Chapter 4. The BRS was again scored in a five-minute post-training assessment period. Wanda was instructed to practice BRT at home and to use it in everyday stressful situations. She was given forms to rate her Subjective Unit of Distress (SUD) least four times daily, and in stressful situations as they occurred.

In her second session a month later, Wanda's success in practicing relaxation and using it to manage stress were discussed. Her CAS decreased to 7 and her GDS-15 to 0, both well within normal range. A five-minute baseline followed by 20 minutes of Upright BRT was conducted as before. A five-minute post-training assessment was then conducted.

Wanda was provided with an audio recording of Upright BRT instructions, and given homework for practicing and using relaxation. She was asked to mail completed homework to the clinic each week. At her request, frequency of SUD ratings was decreased. A one-month follow up was conducted, before which the CAS, GDS-15 and the Abbreviated Acceptability Rating Profile (AARP)[80] were mailed to her for completion.

Figure 6.17 depicts BRS scores during baseline (A1, A2) and Upright BRT (B1, B2) conditions in both the first and second sessions. Percent relaxed scores were low in Baseline and improved markedly with Upright BRT. A decline in relaxed behavior occurred following the hiatus in treatment, but Upright BRT corrected this lapse.

A substantial decline in subjective distress occurred following BRT, with continued downward trend and substantial decline following the first session of BRT (See Figure 6.18). Following session two, and at Wanda's request, SUD ratings were made every other day. During this period, SUD ratings rose slightly and then declined to levels nearly equal to those observed earlier.

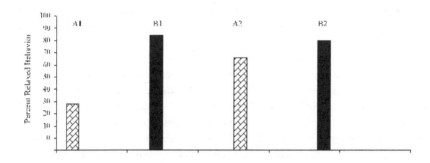

Figure 6.17 Percent upright relaxed behavior across experimental conditions.

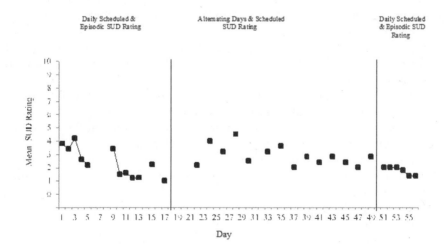

Figure 6.18 Mean SUD rating following Upright Behavioral Relaxation Training (BRT).

ET, anxiety, and depression: Cheryl.

Cheryl, 50 years old, had been diagnosed with ET of the head at age 20. What had been an intermittent problem became more frequent, and she quit her job four years prior to referral because of constant tremor and social anxiety. She also was recently diagnosed with dystonia in her neck, which caused her head to twist to the right, with consequent neck and shoulder pain. She had been prescribed Clonazepam for anxiety and Paroxetine for depression, but stated she wished to decrease medication.

The function-based behavioral interview revealed a number of eliciting and evoking events related to her anxiety and depression, including interactions with her husband and their adult children, and attending social functions. Activities such as vacuuming, sweeping, and computer work exacerbated her dystonia. Her scores on the Clinical Anxiety Scale (CAS) indicated mild clinical anxiety, and on the Geriatric Depression Scale (GDS-15) placed her in the mild-to-moderate range.

A treatment goal of managing stress and the usefulness of relaxation in achieving this was agreed upon. Accordingly, she was taught all ten of the relaxed postures using Reclined BRT procedures. She was asked to make SUD ratings four times daily at home and to practice relaxation at least once a day.

At her second session, Cheryl's SUD data indicated that she engaged in negative self-talk prior to social situations and left early to avoid interacting. She also reported anxiety when she was home alone. She was given proficiency training in Reclined BRT and encouraged to practice daily and to relax whenever she felt anxious.

Cheryl attended therapy twice weekly for two weeks but then her schedule decreased to once or twice a month because of turmoil in her home life. On the sixth session, Upright BRT was introduced and assertiveness training[87] begun to help her deal more effectively with family and other social demands. This continued five more sessions until Cheryl felt confident with her coping skills.

Cheryl acquired relaxation skills quickly, as measured by the BRS, reaching 100 percent relaxed after proficiency training (See Fig. 6.19). There was some decline in performance thereafter but she remained at 80 percent or better. Upright BRT was trained on Session 6, and baseline score on the Upright BRS are shown in this figure. Only one other assessment of Upright BRS was made because the focus changed to assertiveness training and supportive counseling.

Current levels of anxiety and depression were measured each session by the CAS and the GDS-15. Figure 6.20 shows that Cheryl's anxiety scores decreased steadily over the course of BRT, with some variability in subse-

PAIN AND ANXIETY DISORDERS • 185

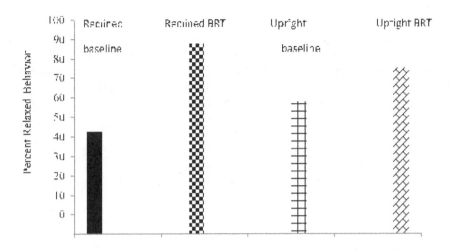

Figure 6.19 Percent relaxed behavior during baseline, reclined and upright relaxed positions.

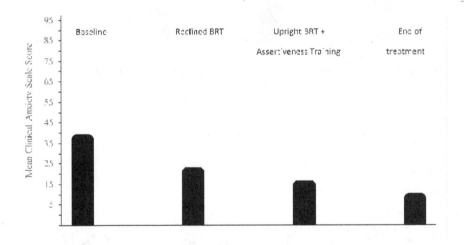

Figure 6.20 Clinical Anxiety Scale (CAS) scores across experimental conditions.

quent sessions as difficult matters relating to her home life were dealt with. Her final scores were well below the cut-off for clinically significant anxiety.

Similarly, her scores on the depression inventory (see Figure 6.21) decreased markedly during BRT and remained at low levels thereafter. Her scores fell within the "normal" range.

186 • CHAPTER 6

Finally, Cheryl's self-ratings of distress, made daily at home on the SUD scale, are shown in Figure 6.22. These represent mean ratings for the period prior to each session. As with the other subjective measures, SUD scores decreased during BRT, and remained at lower levels, with some variability, in later sessions. After one month hiatus, Cheryl scheduled her last visit (end of treatment on Figures 6.18-6.20). At this visit she reported that she was satisfied with the progress she had made. She was willing to record SUD ratings for one week after the visit and mail them in.

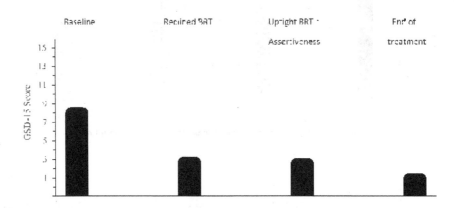

Figure 6.21 Geriatric Depression Scale score across experimental conditions.

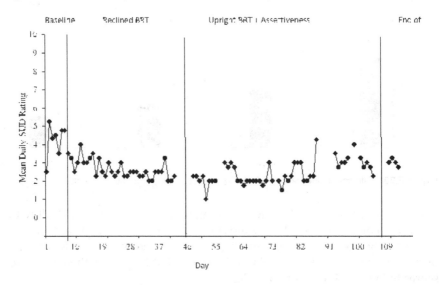

Figure 6.22 Mean daily SUD ratings across experimental conditions.

Summary

Anxiety and stress can significantly impair the quality of life for anyone but this is especially the case for individuals with PD. In each of the cases described, BRT as part of a treatment package resulted in decreases in subjective distress and self-reported anxiety. It is also important to note that for each participant, reclined relaxation was not feasible and training was completed in the upright position. Like reclined BRT, the postures of UBRT are also empirically validated. By acquiring relaxation skills, despite having impaired movement, both participants learned an effective self-management procedure that aided them in coping with stressful events and anxiety.

CONCLUSIONS

This chapter focused on the application of BRT to manage pain and anxiety. The evidence supports the use of BRT across a range of pain disorders, levels of cognitive functioning, types of anxiety, and functional impairment. Lundervold and colleagues[31,32] demonstrated the impact of BRT on pain interference and pain anxiety as part of the Behavioral Activation Treatment for Pain (BAT-P). While Reclined BRT lessened both pain interference and pain anxiety, the implementation of Upright BRT resulted in further reductions in each of these outcome measures. Regular practice of the relaxed postures can reduce general levels of arousal, while engagement in relaxed behavior in upsetting situations provides a coping response that functions as an alternative to further pain, anxiety, and other forms of maladaptive behavior. BRT is an integral element of BAT-P package, and the clinical research protocols do not allow its precise contribution to the overall outcomes to be isolated.

In a similar vein, BRT was shown to be effective in the management of PD-related anxiety.[75,81] BRT is an effective, efficient intervention that can be tailored to the particular needs of individual participants. Moreover, as Tatum et al.[57] demonstrated, BRT can easily be adapted to group instruction. In so doing, group based BRT for participants with chronic pain or health-related anxiety needs to be explored.

REFERENCES

[1]Dahlhamer. J., Lucas, J., Zelaya, C. et al. (2018). Prevalence of chronic pain and high-impact chronic pain among adults–United States, 2016. *Morbity and Mortality Weekly Report, 67*, 1001–1006. doi: http://dx.doi.org/10.15585/mmwr.mm6736a2. Retrieved December 26, 2018 from https://www.cdc.gov/mmwr/volumes/67/wr/mm6736a2.htm.

[2]Kessler, R. C., Chiu, W. T, Demler, O., Merikangas, & K. R., & Walters, E. E. (2005). Prevalence, severity, and comorbidity of 12-month DSM-IV disorders in the National Comorbidity Survey Replication. *Archives of General Psychiatry, 62*(6), 617–27. PMID: 15939839. https://doi.org/10.1001/archpsyc.62.6.617

[3]Headache disorders. Retrieved March 15, 2019 from https://www.who.int/en/news-room/fact-sheets/detail/headache-disorders) 8 April, 2016.

[4]Goadsby, P. J., Holland, P. R., Martins-Oliveira, M., Hoffmann, J., Schankin, C., & Akerman, S. (2017). Pathophysiology of migraine: A disorder of sensory processing. *Physiology Review, 97*(2), 553–622. https://doi.org/10.1152/physrev.00034.2015

[5]Blanchard, E. B., & Andrasik, F. (1985). *Management of chronic headaches*. New York: Pergamon.

[6]Walsh, M., Morrison, T., & McGuire, B. E. (2011). Chronic pain in adults with an intellectual disability: Prevalence, impact and health service use based on caregiver report. *Pain, 152*,1951–1957. doi: 10.1016/j.pain.2011.02.031.

[7]LaChapelle, D. L., Hadjistavropoulos, T., & Kenneth, C. (1999). Pain measurement in persons with intellectual disabilities. *The Clinical Journal of Pain, 15*(1), 13–23. https://doi.org/10.1097/00002508-199903000-00004

[8]Axmon, A., Ahlström, G., & Westergren, W. (2018). Pain and pain medication among older people with intellectual disabilities in comparison with the general population. *Healthcare (Basel), 6*(2), 67. doi: 10.3390/healthcare6020067

[9]Breau, L. M., & Burkitt, C. (2009). Assessing pain in children with intellectual disabilities. *Pain Research and Management, 14*(2), 116–120, 2009. https://doi.org/10.1155/2009/642352.

[10]McGuire, B. E., Daly, P., & Smyth, F. (2010). Chronic pain in people with intellectual disability: Under-recognized and under-treated? *Journal of Intellectual Disability Research, 54*(3), 240–245. https://doi.org/10.1111/j.1365-2788.2010.01254.x

[11]May, M.A., & Kennedy, C.H. (2010). Health and Problems behavior among people with intellectual disabilities. *Behavior Analysis Practice, 3*(2), 4–12. doi: 10.1007/BF03391759

[12]Kennedy, S., O'Higgins, S.O., Sarma, K., Willig, C., & McGuire, E.E. (2014). Evaluation of a group based cognitive behavioral therapy program for menstrual pain management in young women with intellectual disabilities: protocol for a mixed-methods controlled clinical trial. *BMC Womens Health. 14*, 107.

[13]McManus, S., Treacy, M., & McGuire, B. E. (2014). Cognitive behavioral therapy for chronic pain in people with an intellectual disability: a case series using components of the Feeling Better program. *Journal of Intellectual Disabilities Research, 58*(3), 296–306. doi: 10.1111/jir.12018.

[14]Michultka, D., Poppen, R., & Blanchard, E. B. (1988). Relaxation training as a treatment for chronic headaches in an individual having severe developmental disabilities. *Biofeedback and Self-Regulation, 13,* 257–266. https://doi.org/10.1007/BF00999174

[15]Eufemia, R. L., & Wesolowski, M. D. (1983). The use of a new relaxation method in a case of tension headache. *Journal of Behavior Therapy and Experimental Psychiatry, 14,* 355–358. https://doi.org/10.1016/0005-7916(83)90080-0

[16]Giardono, L. (1997). Behavioral relaxation training for neurofacial pain. *Personal communication to the third author.*

[17]Walitt, B., Nahin, R. L., Katz, R. S., Bergman, M. J., & Wolfe, F. (2015). The prevalence and characteristics of fibromyalgia in the 2012 National Health Interview Survey. *PLoS One.* 2015; 10(9): e0138024. https://doi.org/10.1371/journal.pone.0138024

[18]Clauw, D. J., & Chrousos, G. P. (1997). Chronic pain and fatigue syndromes: Overlapping clinical and neuroendocrine features and potential pathogenic mechanisms. *Neuroimmunomodulation, 4,* 134–153. https://doi.org/10.1159/000097332

[19]Kosek, E., Ekholm, J., & Hansson, P. (1996). Sensory dysfunction in fibromyalgia participants with implications for pathogenic mechanisms. *Pain, 57,* 277–292.

[20]White, K. P., Speechley, M., Harth, M., & Ostbye, T. (1995). Fibromyalgia in rheumatology practice: A survey of Canadian rheumatologists. *Journal of Rheumatoloy, 22,* 717–721.

[21]Baumstark, K. E., & Buckelew, S. P. (1992). Fibromyalgia: Clinical signs, research findings, treatment implications and future directions. *Annals of Behavioral Medicine, 14,* 282–291.

[22]McCracken, L. M., & Gross, R. T. (1998). The role of pain-related anxiety reduction in the outcome of multidisciplinary treatment for chronic low back pain: Preliminary results. *Journal of Occupational Rehabilitation, 8,* 179–189. https://doi.org/10.1023/A:1021374322673

[23]McCracken, L. M., Zaylor, C., & Gross, R. T. (1992). The Pain Anxiety Symptom Scale: Development and validation of a scale to measure fear of pain. *Pain, 50,* 67–74. https://doi.org/10.1016/0304-3959(92)90113-P

[24]Kehoe, E. J., & Mcrae, M. (1998). Classical conditioning. In W. O'Donohue (Ed.), *Learning and behavior therapy.* (pp. 36–58). Boston: Allyn and Bacon.

[25]Fordyce, W. E. (1976). *Behavioral methods for chronic pain and illness.* St. Louis: Mosby.

[26]Fordyce, W. E (2000). Learned pain. Pain as behavior. In J. Loeser, S. Butler, C. R., Chapman & D. C. Turk (Eds.), *Bonica's management of pain* (3rd ed., pp. 478–482).

[27]Turk, D. C., Okifuji, A., Starz, T. W., & Sinclair, J. (1996). Interdisciplinary treatment for fibromyalgia syndrome: Clinical and statistical significance. *Arthritis Care and Research, 11,* 186–195. https://doi.org/10.1002/art.1790110306

[28]Jacobson, N. S., Dobson, K. S., Truax, P. A., Addis, M. E., Koerner, K., Gollan, J. K., Prince, S. E. (1996). A component analysis of cognitive-behavioral treatment depression. *Journal of Consulting and Clinical Psychology, 64,* 295–304. https://doi.org/10.1037/0022-006X.64.2.295

[29]Hopko, D. R., Lejuez, C. W., & Hopko, S. D. (2004). Behavioral activation as an intervention for co-existent depressive and anxiety symptoms. *Clinical Case Studies, 3*, 37–48. https://doi.org/10.1177/1534650103258969

[30]Lundervold, D. A., Talley, C., & Buermann, M. (2006). Effect of behavioral activation treatment on fibromyalgia-related pain anxiety cognition. *International Journal of Behavioral Consultation and Therapy, 2*(1), 73–84. https://doi.org/10.1037/h0100768

[31]Lundervold, D. A., Talley, C., & Buermann, M. (2008). Effect of behavioral activation treatment on chronic fibromyalgia pain: Replication and extension. *International Journal of Behavioral Consultation and Therapy, 4*(2), 146–157. https://doi.org/10.1037/h0100839

[32]Ferraro, F. R., & Chelminski, I. (1996). Preliminary data on the Geriatric Depression Scale-Short Form (GDS-SF) in a young adult sample. *Journal of Clinical Psychology, 52*, 443–447. https://doi.org/10.1002/(SICI)1097-4679(199607)52:4<443:AID-JCLP9>3.0.CO;2-Q

[33]Herrnstein, R. J. (1961). Relative and absolute strength of response as a function of frequency of reinforcement. *Journal of the Experimental Analysis of Behavior, 4*, 267–272. https://doi.org/10.1901/jeab.1961.4-267

[34]Wolpe, J. (1958). *Psychotherapy by reciprocal inhibition*. Palo Alto, CA: Stanford University Press.

[35]Poppen, R. (1995). *Joseph Wolpe*. Thousand Oaks, CA: Sage Publications, Inc.

[36]Helfer, S. L. (1984). *Systematic desensitization with behavioral relaxation training: Assessment of cognitive, physiological, and behavioral response systems*. Unpublished master's thesis, Southern Illinois University at Carbondale.

[37]Wolpe, J., & Lang, P. J. (1964). A fear survey schedule for use in behavior therapy. *Behavior Research and Therapy, 2*, 27-30. https://doi.org/10.1016/0005-7967(64)90051-8

[38]Jones, L. C., Mrug, S., Elliott, M. N., Toomey, S. L., Tortolero, S., & Schuster, M. A. (2017). Chronic physical health conditions and emotional problems from early adolescence through mid-adolescence. *Academy of Pediatrics, 17*(6), 649–655. doi: 10.1016/j.acap.2017.02.002

[39]Vrijens, D., Berghmans, B. Nieman, F. van Os, J, van Koeveringe, G., & Leue, C. (2017). Prevalence of anxiety and depressive symptoms and their association with pelvic floor dysfunctions: A cross sectional cohort study at a Pelvic Care Centre. *Neurourology and Urodynamics, 36*(7),1816–1823. doi: 10.1002/nau.23186.

[40]Tang, W. K., Lau, C. G., Mok, V., Ungvari, G. S., & Wong, K. S. (2013). Impact of anxiety on health-related quality of life after stroke: a cross-sectional study. *Archives of Physical Medicine and Rehabilitation, 94*(12), 2535–41. doi: 10.1016/j.apmr.2013.07.012.)

[41]Potvin, O., Forget, H., Grenier, S., Préville, M., & Hudon, C. (2011). Anxiety, depression, and 1-year incident cognitive impairment in community-dwelling older adults. *Journal of the American Geriatric Society, 59*(8), 1421–8. doi: 10.1111/j.1532-5415.2011.03521.x.

[42]Hwang, T. J., Masterman, D. L., Ortiz, F., Fairbanks, L. A., & Cummings, J. L. (2004). Mild cognitive impairment is associated with characteristic neuropsychiatric symptoms. *Alzheimer Disease and Associated Disorders, 18*(1), 17–21. https://doi.org/10.1097/00002093-200401000-00004

[43]Apostolova, L. G., & Cummings J. L. (2008). Neuropsychiatric manifestations in mild cognitive impairment: A systematic review of the literature. *Dementia and Geriatric Cognitive Disorders, 8*(25), 115–126. doi:10.1159/000112509

[44]Lundervold, D. A., & Holt, P. S. (2011). *Brief imaginal exposure for specific phobia with an older adult with mild cognitive impairment (MCI) with amnesia.* Anxiety and Depression Association of America, San Jose, CA.

[45]Lundervold, D. A., Holt, P. S., Beasley, B. W., & Pahwa, R. (2019). *A perfect storm of opportunity: Integrated health care, evidence-based practice and single case research design.* Unpublished manuscript.

[46]Segool, N.K., Carlson, J.S., Goforth, A.N., von der Embse, N., & Barterian, J.A. (2013). Heightened test anxiety among young children: Elementary school students' responses to high stakes testing. *Psychology in the Schools, 50*(5), 489–499. https://doi.org/10.1002/pits.21689

[47]von der Embse, N., & Hasson, R. (2011). Test anxiety and high-stakes test performance between school settings: Implications for educators. *Preventing School Failure: Alternative Education for Children and Youth, 56*(3), 180–187. doi: 10.1080/1045988X.2011.633285

[48]Carey, J., & Dimmitt, C. (2008). A model for evidence-based elementary school counseling: Using school data, research, and evaluation to enhance practice. *The Elementary School Journal, 108*, 422–430. https://doi.org/10.1086/589471

[49]Brott, P. (2006). Counselor education accountability: Training the effective professional school counselor. *Professional School Counseling, 10*, 179–188. https://doi.org/10.5330/prsc.10.2.d61g0v3738863652

[50]Walker, H. M. (2004). Commentary: Use of evidence-based interventions: Where we've been, where we are, and where we need to go. *School Psychology Review, 33*(3) 398-407.

[51]Compton, S., March, J. S., Brent, D., Albano, A. M., Weersing, V. R., & Curry, J. (2004). Cognitive-behavioral psychotherapy for anxiety and depressive disorders in children and adolescents: an evidence-based medicine review. *Journal of the American Academy of Child and Adolescent Psychiatry, 43*(8), 930–59. https://doi.org/10.1097/01.chi.0000127589.57468.bf

[52]Borkovec, T. D., Newman, M. G., Pincus, A. L., & Lytle, R. (2002). A component analysis of cognitive-behavioral therapy for generalized anxiety disorder and the role of interpersonal problems. *Journal of Consulting and Clinical Psychology, 70*, 288–298. doi:10.1037/0022-006X.70.2.288

[53]Rashid, Z. M., & Paris. T. S. (1998). The effects of two types of relaxation training on students' levels of anxiety. *Adolescence, 33*, 129, 99–101.

[54]Spielberger, C. D., Gorsuch, R.L., & Lushene, R. E. (1970). *The State-Trait Anxiety Inventory (STAI) test manual for Form X*. Palo Alto, CA: Consulting Psychologists Press.

[55]Chapell, M. S., Blanding, Z. B., Silverstein, B., Takahashi, M., Newman, B., Gubi, A., & McCann, N. (2005). Test anxiety and academic performance in undergraduate and graduate students. *Journal of Educational Psychology, 97*, 268–274. https://doi.org/10.1037/0022-0663.97.2.268

[56]Tatum, T., Lundervold, D. A., & Ament, P. A. (2006). Abbreviated Upright Behavioral Relaxation Training for test anxiety among college students: Initial results. *International Journal of Behavioral Consultation and Therapy, 2*(4), 475–479. https://doi.org/10.1037/h0101001

[57]Hopko, D., Mahadevan, R., Bare, R., & Hunt, M. K. (2003). The abbreviated math anxiety scale (AMAS). Construction, validity, and reliability. *Assessment, 10*, 178–182. https://doi.org/10.1177/1073191103010002008

[58]Ellgring, H., Seiler, S., Perleth, B., Frings, W. et al. (1993). Psychosocial aspects of Parkinson's disease. *Neurology, 43*(12), Suppl 6, S41–S44.

[59]Louis, E. D., & Machado, D. G. (2015). Tremor-related quality of life: A comparison of essential tremor vs. Parkinson's disease participants. *Parkinsonism & Related Disorders, 21*, 729–735. https://doi.org/10.1016/j.parkreldis.2015.04.019

[60]Gündel, H., Wolf, A., Xidara,V., Busch, R., & Ceballos-Baumann, A. O. (2001). Social phobia in spasmodic torticollis. *Journal of Neurology, Neurosurgery & Psychiatry, 71*, 499–504. https://doi.org/10.1136/jnnp.71.4.499

[61]Garlovsky, J. K., Overton, P. G., & Simpson, J. (2016). Psychological predictors of anxiety and depression in Parkinson's disease: A systematic review. *Journal of Clinical Psychology, 72*(10), 979–998. doi: 10.1002/jclp.22308.

[62]Musacchio, T. Purrer, V., Papagianni, A., Fleischer, A., Mackenrodt, D., Malsch, C., Gelbrich, G., Steigerwald,F., Volkmann, J., & Klebe, S. (2016). Non-motor symptoms of essential tremor are independent of tremor severity and have an impact on quality of life. *Tremor and Other Hyperkinetic Movement Disorders (N Y). 2016 Mar 8;6:361.* doi: 10.7916/D8542NCH

[63]Dissanayaka, N. N, White, E., O'Sullivan, J. D., Marsh, R., Pachana, N. A., & Byrne, G. J. (2014). The clinical spectrum of anxiety in Parkinson's disease. *Movement Disorders, 29*, (8),967–75. doi: 10.1002/mds.25937.

[64]O'Sullivan, S. S., Williams, D. R., & Gallager, D. A. (2008). Nonmotor symptoms as presenting complaints in Parkinson's disease. *Movement Disorders, 23*, 101–106.69.

[65]Wenzel, T., Schnider, P., Wimmer, A., Steinhoff, N., Moraru, E., & Auff, E. (1998). Psychiatric comorbidity in participants with spasmodic torticollis. *Journal of Psychosomatic Research, 44*, 687–690. https://doi.org/10.1016/S0022-3999(97)00229-8

[66]Schneier, F. R., Barnes, L. F., Albert, S. M., & Louis, E. D. (2001). Characteristics of social phobia among persons with essential tremor. *The Journal of Clinical Psychiatry, 62*(5), 367–372. https://doi.org/10.4088/JCP.v62n0511

[67]Lundervold, D. A., Ament, P. A., & Holt, P. (2013). Social anxiety, tremor severity, and tremor disability: A search for clinically relevant measures. *Psychiatry Journal Volume 2013, Article ID 257459, 5 pages* http://dx.doi.org/10.1155/2013/257459

[68]Rutten, S., van der Ven, P. M., Weintraub, D., Pontone, G. M., Leentjens, A. F. G., Berendse, H. W., van der Werf, Y. D., & van den Heuvel, O. A. (2017). Predictors of anxiety in early-stage Parkinson's disease—Results from the first two years of a

prospective cohort study. *Parkinsonism & Related Disorders, 43,* 49–55. https://doi.org/10.1016/j.parkreldis.2017.06.024

[69]Dissanayaka, N. W. (2010). Anxiety disorders in Parkinson's disease: Prevalence and risk factors. *Movement Disorders, 25*(7), 838–845. https://doi.org/10.1002/mds.22833

[70]Dissanayaka, N. W., White, E., O'Sullivan, J. D., Marsh, R., Pachana, N. A., & Byrne, G. J. (2014). The clinical spectrum of anxiety in Parkinson's disease. *Movement Disorders, 29,* 8, 967–975. https://doi.org/10.1002/mds.25937

[71]Chung, W., Poppen, R., & Lundervold, D. A. (1995). Behavioral relaxation training for tremor disorders in older adults. *Biofeedback and Self-Regulation, 20,* 123–135. https://doi.org/10.1007/BF01720969

[72]Schlesinger, I., Benyakov, O., Erikh, I., & Nassar, M. (2014). Relaxation guided imagery reduces motor fluctuations in Parkinson's disease. *Journal of Parkinson's Disease, 4*(3), 431–436. doi: 10.3233/JPD-130338.

[73]Schlesinger, I., Benyakov, O., Erikh, I., Suraiya. S., & Schiller Y. (2009). Parkinson's disease tremor is diminished with relaxation guided imagery. *Movement Disorders, 24*(14), 2059–2062. doi: 10.1002/mds.22671.

[74]Ajimsha, M. S., Majeed, N. A., Chinnavan, E., & Thulasyammal, R. P. (2014). Effectiveness of autogenic training in improving motor performances in Parkinson's disease. *Complementary Therapy and Medicine, 22*(3), 419–425. doi: 10.1016/j.ctim.2014.03.013

[75]Lundervold, D. A., Pahwa, R., & Lyons, K. E. (2013). Behavioral Relaxation Training for Parkinson's Disease related dyskinesia and comorbid social anxiety. *International Journal of Behavioral Consultation and Therapy, 7*(4), 1–5. https://doi.org/10.1037/h0100957

[76]Fahn S., Elton, R. L., & UPDRS program members. Unified Parkinson's Disease Rating Scale. (1987). In S. Fahn, C.D. Marsden, M. Goldstein, & D.B. Calne, (Eds.), *Recent developments in Parkinson's disease, 2* (pp. 153–163). Florham Park, NJ: Macmillan Healthcare Information.

[77]Yesavage, J. A., Brink, T. L., Rose, T. L., Lum, O. Huang, V., Adey, M., & Leirer, V. O. (1983). Development and validation of a geriatric depression screening scale: A preliminary report. *Journal of Psychiatric Research, 17,* 37–49. https://doi.org/10.1016/0022-3956(82)90033-4

[78]Thyer, B. A., & Westhuis, D. (1989). Test-retest reliability of the Clinical Anxiety Scale. *Phobia Practice and Research, 2,* 111–113. https://doi.org/10.1037/t10565-000

[79]Carr, E. G., & Smith, C. E. (1995). Biological setting events for self-injury. *Mental Retardation and Developmental Disabilities Research Reviews, 1*(2), 94–98. https://doi.org/10.1002/mrdd.1410010204

[80]Tarnowski, K. J., & Simonian, S. J. (1992). Assessing treatment acceptance: The abbreviated treatment acceptability rating profile. *Journal of Behavior Therapy and Experimental Psychiatry, 23,* 101–106. https://doi.org/10.1016/0005-7916(92)90007-6

[81]Lundervold, D.A., Pahwa, R., & Lyons, K.E. (2009). Effect of Behavioral Relaxation Training on comorbid general anxiety disorder and Parkinson's disease. *Clinical Gerontologist, 32,* 104–117. https://doi.org/10.1080/07317110802468736

[82]Thanvi, B., Lo, N., & Robinson, T. (2007). Levodopa-induced dyskinesia in Parkinson's disease: clinical features, pathogenesis, prevention and treatment. *Postgraduate Medical Journal, 83*(980), 384–388. doi: 10.1136/pgmj.2006.054759

[83]Tarlow, K. R. (2017). An improved rank correlation effect size statistic for single-case designs: Baseline Corrected Tau. *Behavior Modification, 41*(4), 427–467. http://dx.doi.org/10.1177/0145445516676750

[84]*Baseline corrected tau/Kevin Tarlow*. Retrieved November 13, 2019 from http://ktarlow.com/stats/tau/.

Supplement
Behavior Analyst Certification Board 5th Edition Task List

A. Philosophical Underpinnings
A-1 Identify the goals of behavior analysis as a science (i.e., description, prediction, control).
A-2 Explain the philosophical assumptions underlying the science of behavior analysis (e.g., selectionism, determinism, empiricism, parsimony, pragmatism).
A-3 Describe and explain behavior from the perspective of radical behaviorism.
A-4 Distinguish among behaviorism, the experimental analysis of behavior, applied behavior analysis, and professional practice guided by the science of behavior analysis.
A-5 Describe and define the dimensions of applied behavior analysis (Baer, Wolf, & Risley, (1968).

B. Concepts and Principles
B-1 Define and provide examples of behavior, response, and response class.
B-2 Define and provide examples of stimulus and stimulus class.
B-3 Define and provide examples of respondent and operant conditioning.
B-4 Define and provide examples of positive and negative reinforcement contingencies.
B-5 Define and provide examples of schedules of reinforcement.
B-10 Define and provide examples of stimulus control.

C. Measurement, Data Display, and Interpretation
C-1 Establish operational definitions of behavior.
C-2 Distinguish among direct, indirect, and product measures of behavior.
C-3 Measure occurrence (e.g., frequency, rate, percentage).
C-5 Measure form and strength of behavior (e.g., topography, magnitude).
C-6 Measure trials to criterion.
C-7 Design and implement sampling procedures (i.e., interval recording, time sampling).
C-8 Evaluate the validity and reliability of measurement procedures.

C-9   Select a measurement system to obtain representative data given the dimensions of behavior and the logistics of observing and recording.
C-10 Graph data to communicate relevant quantitative relations (e.g., equal-interval graphs, bar graphs, cumulative records).
C-11 Interpret graphed data.

D. Experimental Design
D-1   Distinguish between dependent and independent variables.
D-5   Use single-subject experimental designs (e.g., reversal, multiple baseline, multielement, changing criterion).

G. Behavior-Change Procedures
G-1   Use positive and negative reinforcement procedures to strengthen behavior.
G-5   Use modeling and imitation training.
G-6   Use instructions and rules.
G-9   Use discrete-trial, free-operant, and naturalistic teaching arrangements.
G-14 Use reinforcement procedures to weaken behavior (e.g., DRA, FCT, DRO, DRL, NCR).
G-20 Use self-management strategies.

H. Selecting and Implementing Interventions
H-1   State intervention goals in observable and measurable terms.
H-4   When a target behavior is to be decreased, select an acceptable alternative behavior to be established or increased.
H-6   Monitor client progress and treatment integrity.
H-7   Make data-based decisions about the effectiveness of the intervention and the need for treatment revision.
H-9   Collaborate with others who support and/or provide services to clients.

Chapter 7
Neurological Diseases and Disorders

Diseases of and injuries to the brain, spine, and nerves form the basis of neurological disorders. The illness or disorder can affect the entire nervous system or a single neuron. The disorders may involve the central, peripheral, or autonomic nervous system. Classification of neurological disorders is based on the location, dysfunction, or cause, and the disorder may have a chronic, relapsing, or remitting course. With improved health care and nutrition, many individuals, who in earlier times would have succumbed to a neurological insult, live with the biobehavioral sequelae of an impaired nervous system. It is readily apparent that neurological disorders affect performance of instrumental activities of daily living, limit social interactions, and are related to significant emotional distress.

ESSENTIAL TREMOR

Essential tremor (ET), the most common movement disorder, has peak incidence in later life although it sometimes affects younger adults.[1] ET is a complex syndrome with multiple neurologic causal pathways and, possibly, is a family of diseases.[2] While most patients have *kinetic (action) tremor* (rhythmic oscillation of the hand during intentional movement), they may also suffer from *resting tremor* (limb or hand is supported), *postural tremor* (limb held against gravity), or *voice tremor*. Medication poorly controls ET, does not alter emotional distress, and has been described as a trial and error process of treatment. No consistent pharmacologic benefit has been observed.[3]

ET is exacerbated by emotional arousal, stress, fatigue, and observation by others. ET significantly impairs performance of activities of daily living (ADL), social interactions, and emotional well-being.[4,5] About one-third of individuals with ET also suffer from social anxiety disorder.[6,7] Lundervold and colleagues[7] found that subjective unit of distress ratings (SUD) in specific situations, and social phobia scale[8] scores, were related to tremor disability in the form of impaired performance of ADL. A large-scale (N = 1,418) survey[9] of the needs of ET patients revealed that 48 percent reported that neurologists are not addressing the psychological effects of ET, including nonpharmacological interventions for stress, anxiety, and movement problems.

Effects of BRT on Essential Tremor

Chung, Poppen, and Lundervold[10] employed BRT with two older adults with movement disorders; one with ET, the second with Parkinson's Disease (PD). The first case is described here. Mr. D, an 86-year-old man, reported tremor onset at age 16. He was diagnosed with ET by a neurologist later in life. While mild in severity, both postural and kinetic tremor interfered with ADLs such as eating, drinking, and dressing. Mr. D lived alone and participated in community senior citizen activities. He took 230 milligrams of primidone for ET daily throughout the study.

An extended A-B multiphase design was employed, consisting of baseline (four sessions), reclined BRT (eight sessions), and upright BRT (four sessions). A follow-up session was conducted two weeks after final training. Sessions were conducted once or twice weekly. BRT was conducted for 15 to 20 minutes, followed by a five-minute post-training BRS observation period. Transfer of training from the reclined to upright position was assessed in four sessions during the reclined BRT phase. After reaching criterion of at least 85 percent relaxed in the reclined position for three consecutive sessions, upright BRT commenced with the same criterion. Throughout the BRT phases, Mr. D was instructed to practice relaxation at home every day for at least 15 minutes.

Postural tremor for both right and left hands was assessed at the end of each BRS observation period by asking Mr. D, while seated, to extend his arm slowly in front, with wrist extended and hand open, and to maintain this position for 20 seconds. Kinetic tremor was assessed by asking him to extend his right and left arms as before, to touch his nose with extended forefinger, and to return to rest. Tremor during these actions was rated using the Clinical Rating of Tremor scale (CRTS).[11] Mr. D rated his own tremor within each session and was given a self-rating sheet for tremor severity that targeted activities of eating, drinking, and dressing at home. To determine if tremor was related to tension in muscles controlling the affected limb, EMG levels in the forearm flexor and extensor muscles were recorded concurrently with tremor assessment.

Figure 7.1 shows BRS scores (percent relaxed) in both reclined and upright positions across conditions. Mr. D rapidly learned the relaxed pos-

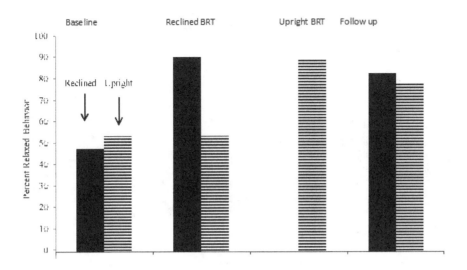

Figure 7.1 Percent relaxed behavior in the reclined and upright positions across experimental conditions for an older adult man with essential tremor.

Based on Chung, W., Poppen, R., & Lundervold, D. A. (1995). Behavioral relaxation training for tremor disorders in older adults. *Biofeedback and Self-Regulation, 20*(2), 123–135.

tures, achieving 80 percent during the first BRT session. He required several more sessions to reach the 85 percent criterion and achieved nearly 100 percent in the last session. No transfer of training from reclined to upright relaxed positions was observed; he remained at around 50 percent relaxed until Upright BRT was given, at which time he rapidly attained criterion performance. BRS scores remained about 80 percent relaxed for both reclined and upright BRT at follow-up.

Clinical ratings of tremor severity scores for both postural and kinetic tremor showed marked improvement after BRT. Mean values for each phase are given in Figure 7.2A. Baseline scores were in the "mild" to "moderate" range and decreased to the "mild" or "no tremor" range, with several zero scores, in reclined BRT, upright BRT, and follow-up sessions. Tremor tended to be slightly greater in his right (dominant) hand as compared to his left.

Mean forearm EMG levels during postural and kinetic assessment, across phases, are shown in Figure 7.2B. With relaxation training, muscle tension decreased to very low levels in both right and left arms, though were slightly higher on the right. Mr. D rated his tremor during eating every day at home. Mean self-ratings across conditions are shown in Figure 7.3. These showed great improvement, falling to zero levels at follow-up.

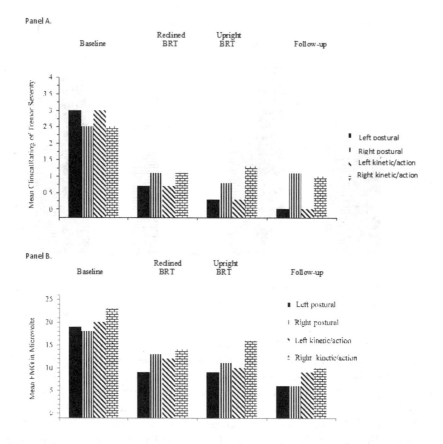

Figure 7.2 Panel A. Mean EMG of right and left forearm extensor and clinical ratings of tremor severity (Panel B) during repeated kinetic (nose touch) and postural (arm extension) clinical tremor assessment across experimental conditions.

In Chung, W., Poppen, R., & Lundervold, D. A. (1995). Behavioral relaxation training for tremor disorders in older adults. *Biofeedback and Self-Regulation, 20*(2), 123–135.

This case study demonstrated that an older person with ET can learn relaxed postures and reduce clinical and self-ratings of tremor, as well as forearm EMG levels, during postural and kinetic assessments of tremor. He reported this tremor reduction transferred to his daily living activity of eating.

BRT for Tremor Related to Activities of Daily Living

Lundervold, Belwood, Craney, and Poppen[12] conducted a systematic replication of the above study, in which tremor was measured while participants

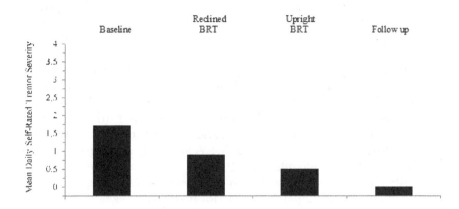

Figure 7.3 Mean daily self-rated tremor severity during eating across experimental conditions for an older adult man with essential tremor.

Based on Chung, W., Poppen, R., & Lundervold, D. A. (1995). Behavioral relaxation training for tremor disorders in older adults. *Biofeedback and Self-Regulation*, 20(2), 123–135.

Table 7.1
Participant Characteristics

Participant	Age	Tremor Type	Severity		Duration	GDS	MSQ	Medication
			Right	Left				
Carlos	73	Kinetic	4	3	4 years	3	9	None
		Postural	5	2				
		Resting	0	0				
Nora	83	Kinetic	4	5	15 years	3	9	10 mg propranolol t.i.d.
		Postural	7	7				
		Resting	0	0				

Based on Lundervold et al. (1999). Reduction of tremor severity and disability following behavioral relaxation training. *Journal of Behavior Therapy and Experimental Psychiatry*, 30, 119–135.

engaged in activities of daily living (ADL), namely eating or drinking. Two older adults with ET, described in Table 7.1, participated.

Relaxation training and assessment proceeded similarly to Chung et al. After baseline assessment, reclined BRT was administered to a criterion of at least 80 percent relaxed on the BRS for three consecutive sessions, followed by Upright BRT to the same criterion. After each BRS scoring period, EMG was recorded while participants engaged in simulated ADL tasks of eating and/or drinking while seated upright at a table. Eating consisted of scooping a spoonful of dry cereal from a bowl, bringing it to the lips, and returning it to the bowl. Drinking consisted of bringing a cupful of hot water to the lips and returning it to the table. No food or liquid was actually ingested. Each task lasted approximately two minutes, was performed with both right and left hands, and was recorded on video. Tremor severity was scored using Bain's[13] 10-point clinical rating scale based on the video recording after the session. Participants self-rated their tremor immediately after the tasks. Carlos engaged only in eating, and Nora in both eating and drinking. Participants were asked to practice relaxation at home and to make daily ratings of their tremor related to eating and drinking. A follow-up assessment occurred seven weeks after the final relaxation training session. Inter-rater agreement on the BRS and CRTS was determined on approximately one-quarter of the sessions. Reliability averaged 90 percent for both measures.

Both participants learned to relax using BRT, achieving the 80 percent criterion during reclined training, but reaching only 75 percent during upright training, as shown in Figure 7.4. Performance declined at follow-up, falling to baseline levels for upright BRS, although retaining almost 75 percent of the reclined postures. Participants reported that they did not practice relaxation during the interim since the last training session.

Within-session clinician (CRTS) and self-ratings of tremor severity (SRTS) during performance of the ADL tasks, and daily self-ratings at home, are shown in Figure 7.5. Carlos had high levels of tremor severity during the

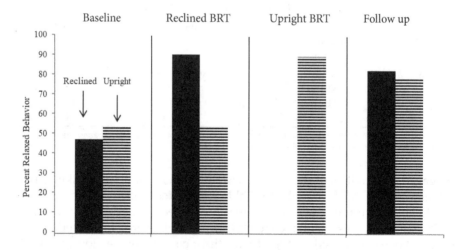

Figure 7.4 Mean Behavioral Relaxation Scale (BRS) scores for Carlos and Nora across experimental conditions.

Based on Lundervold et al. (1999). Reduction of tremor severity and disability following behavioral relaxation training. *Journal of Behavior Therapy and Experimental Psychiatry, 30*, 119–135.

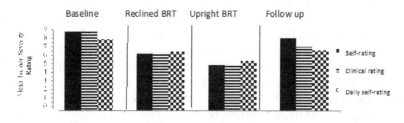
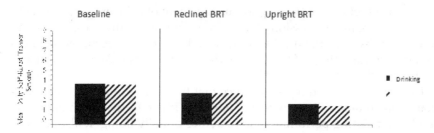

Figure 7.5
Based on Lundervold et al. (1999). Reduction of tremor severity and disability following behavioral relaxation training. *Journal of Behavior Therapy and Experimental Psychiatry, 30*, 119–135.

eating task (Figure 7.5A). Clinician ratings were consistent with self-ratings. Tremor ratings declined during reclined BRT, and further improvements occurred with upright BRT. However, tremor ratings returned to baseline levels at follow-up; an unplanned reversal which we attribute to lack of relaxation practice.

Statistical analysis of single-subject data is helpful in determining the significance of observed trends. Such analyses require ruling out autocorrelation among error terms in the data set. This rationale is detailed in Lundervold et al.[12] and Lundervold and Poppen.[14] Analysis of variance (ANOVA) of Carlos' SRTS data showed significant decreases in both relaxation conditions as compared to baseline. Similar results were found for clinical ratings (CRTS). Daily ratings of tremor severity made by Carlos and his wife indicated a slight decline in tremor severity following reclined BRT, with further diminution of severity in the upright BRT phase. But autocorrelation in the daily rating data prevented statistical evaluation of these changes.

Nora displayed mild tremor during baseline in both the eating and drinking tasks, as shown in Figure 7.5B and C. Self- and clinician-ratings appear consistent with each other. SRTS declined to very low levels during relaxation training, with lowest levels during the upright phase. As with Carlos, there was a return to baseline at follow-up. Statistical analyses showed the decreases in the two BRT conditions, as compared to baseline, were beyond chance for both SRTS and CRTS measures. Nora did not complete daily ratings at home.

EMG levels were recorded from several muscle sites (forearm flexors and extensors, biceps, and deltoids) while the participants performed the ADL tasks. However, no consistent relationships between EMG values and task performance, tremor severity, or phase of the study were found for either participant.

Lundervold et al.[12] also calculated a cost-benefit ratio for the clinical application of relaxation training for management of ET. Compared to medication, nine treatment sessions (one assessment, eight BRT sessions) were more expensive than medication; however, the 47 to 66 percent reduction in self- and clinical ratings of tremor severity and improved ADL performance offset the initial cost.

This study provided more evidence that BRT is useful in teaching relaxation skills to older adults with ET, and that it is effective in ameliorating their tremor during performance of activities of daily living. It also demonstrated the importance of regular practice to maintain relaxation benefits. The relationship between tremor and muscle tension was not established in this study; this inconsistency has been noted by others.[15] Because of this, a multibehavior-multimethod measurement approach using direct observation and self-report is important. The findings also suggested that relaxation training may be useful in a stepped-care treatment model for ET, with relaxation training being the first step.

BRT and EMG Biofeedback for Tremor Related to ADL

Lundervold and Poppen[14] extended the previous research to include a dynamic EMG biofeedback component, in addition to relaxation, to address

Table 7.2
Participant Characteristics

Participant	Age	Tremor Type	Severity		Duration	GDS	MSQ	Medication
			Right	Left				
ED	51	Kinetic	3	2	36 years	4	9	None
		Postural	0	2				
		Resting	0	0				
TH	77	Kinetic	3	2	20 years	3	9	None
		Postural	7	7				
		Resting	0	0				
MA	83	Kinetic	4	N/A	65 years	0	9	10 mg Inderol daily
		Postural	7	N/A				
		Resting	0	0				

Based on Lundervold et al. (1999). Reduction of tremor severity and disability following behavioral relaxation training. *Journal of Behavior Therapy and Experimental Psychiatry, 30,* 119–135.

tremor that occurs while engaging in eating or drinking ADL tasks. Participants included one man and two women who had been diagnosed with ET. The focus was on kinetic tremor, although they displayed postural or resting tremor as well. Participant details are shown in Table 7.2.

Tremor was assessed while the person engaged in two-minute simulated eating or drinking tasks, as described previously. Assessments were conducted both pre- and post-relaxation within each session. ADL performance was video recorded and later scored using the Bain rating scale. Participants self-rated their tremor on an analogous scale after completion of each task. They also used this scale to make daily home ratings of tremor while eating or drinking. In addition, EMG levels of forearm flexor and extensor muscles were recorded during relaxation and ADL performance. Relaxation was measured by scoring the BRS, either reclined or upright as appropriate, during five-minute observation periods following baseline and training relaxation sessions. Reliability of BRS and CRTS observations were established as in the previous studies.

After initial screening, intervention occurred in four phases: baseline, reclined BRT, upright BRT, and dynamic EMG biofeedback. A follow-up session was conducted 12 weeks after the end of treatment. During baseline, participants were asked to relax as they ordinarily would, in both a reclining and an upright chair. Baseline continued to a criterion of no more than ten percent variation in reclined BRS scores over three sessions. Reclined BRT was administered in the usual fashion to a criterion of at least 80 percent relaxed on the BRS for three consecutive sessions. Upright BRT was then administered to the same criterion. In the dynamic biofeedback phase, an auditory signal proportional to muscle activity was provided while the participant engaged in the ADL tasks for durations between 10 and 20 minutes. During biofeedback, ED was trained to reduce forearm extensor tension while engaged in both drinking and eating. TH was trained to reduce extensor tension during eating. MA was trained to increase bicep tension during drinking in an effort to stabilize her upper arm.

Figure 7.6 shows that two of the three participants, ED and MA, reached the acquisition criterion on the BRS in the reclined and upright positions. BRS scores for TH improved somewhat but did not reach criterion due to the severity of her tremor, as well as myoclonic jerks, during the post-training observation period. At follow-up, for ED and TH, reclined and upright BRS scores decreased, but remained above baseline levels. MA maintained the relaxed postures at criterion levels for both positions.

ED's within-session self-rated tremor during ADL tasks, pre- and post-relaxation, are shown in Figure 7.7 and Table 7.3. When BRT was implemented, post-training SRTS scores decreased markedly, compared to pre-training, for both the eating and drinking tasks. Post-training SRTS also decreased in successive experimental phases, with some apparent increase at follow-up, though still below baseline levels. Statistical analyses of ED's SRTS data showed the within-session effect to be highly significant, and that tremor was lower in treatment phases as compared to baseline. Because only one follow-up session occurred, there were insufficient data to include in the analysis.

Clinical ratings of ED's tremor while performing ADL tasks show the same pattern as his self-ratings, though were generally lower. CRTS scores significantly decreased during the relaxation and biofeedback phases, as compared to baseline, but showed no differences between treatment conditions.

ED and his wife also completed daily ratings of tremor severity for eating and drinking. ED reported a decline in daily ratings during upright and dynamic biofeedback phases, which were maintained at follow up assessment. Mrs. ED's ratings generally paralleled her husband's, though she reported a decline in tremor severity during reclined BRT (see Table 7.3). However, autocorrelation in these data precluded statistical evaluation of these changes.

EMG data for ED's forearm extensor muscles, for which he received training in the dynamic biofeedback phase, could not be evaluated because of autocorrelation. However, analysis of his flexor EMG was possible. For this muscle, significant reductions in the post- as compared to pre-relaxation assessments was found. And flexor EMG was lower in the relaxation and biofeedback

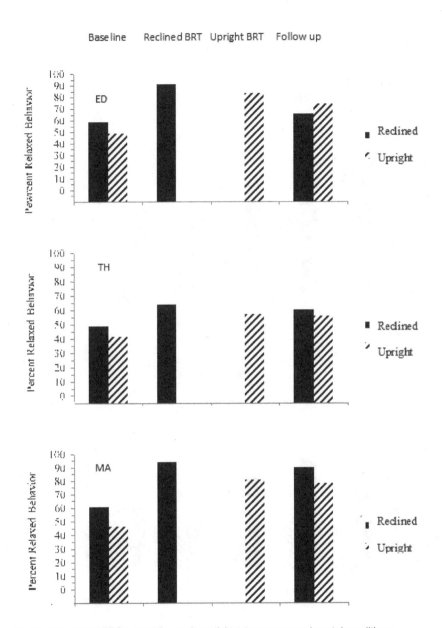

Figure 7.6 Mean BRS scores for each participant across experimental conditions.
Based on Lundervold, D. A. & Poppen, R. (2004). Biobehavioral intervention for older adults coping with essential tremor. *Applied Psychophysiology and Biofeedback, 29*, 63–74.

Panel A. Eating.

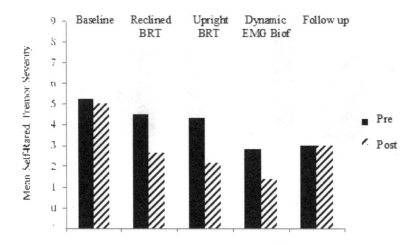

Panel B. Drinking.

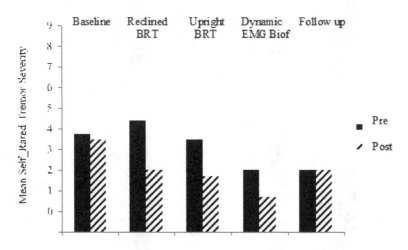

Figure 7.7 ED's within session mean pre-post training self-rating of tremor severity right hand eating (Panel A) and drinking from a cup (Panel B) across experimental conditions.

Based on Lundervold, D. A. & Poppen, R. (2004). Biobehavioral intervention for older adults coping with essential tremor. *Applied Psychophysiology and Biofeedback*, 29, 63–74.

Table 7.3
Mean daily self-ratings of tremor severity during eating and drinking

Participant		Baseline	Reclined	Upright BRT	Reclined EMG Biofeedback	Follow Up
Ed	Eating	3.19	3.15	2.17	-----	1.57
Mrs. Ed		2.54	1.64	1.00	-----	1.14
Ed	Drinking	3.25	3.06	1.78	-----	1.43
Mrs. Ed		2.69	1.64	.89	-----	1.00
TH	Eating	4.65	4.86	3.95	-----	1.00
MA	Drinking	3.51	2.34	1.36	1.31	1.43

Based on Lundervold, D. A. & Poppen, R. (2004). Biobehavioral intervention for older adults coping with essential tremor. *Applied Psychophysiology and Biofeedback, 29,* 63–74.

conditions, as compared to baseline, with no differences between treatment phases. Similar results were found in both the eating and drinking tasks.

TH reported the most severe tremor of the three participants, and was able to achieve the least degree of relaxation during training (Figure 7.6). However, as seen in Figure 7.8, when BRT was implemented, she experienced decreased tremor during post-training assessment as compared to pre-training, and showed progressive decreases over treatment phases. Her improvement was maintained and even enhanced at follow-up. Clinical ratings of her tremor were somewhat less severe, but showed the same pattern of change over the course of treatment. Statistical analyses of tremor ratings, both SRTS and CRTS, showed significant reductions in the treatment phases, as compared to baseline, with no difference between treatments.

TH's daily home ratings of tremor severity when eating, as shown in Table 7.3, appeared to decrease when BRT was implemented, and to further diminish during the dynamic biofeedback phase. However, autocorrelation in these data proscribed statistical analysis.

TH's forearm extensor EMG, measured while performing the eating task, decreased when reclined BRT was implemented, and remained at these lower levels in the subsequent upright BRT and dynamic biofeedback stages. Similar results were obtained for her forearm flexor muscles. Statistical analyses showed significant differences between baseline and treatment conditions, with no differences between treatments, for both EMG placements.

MA rated her tremor in the low moderate range prior to treatment (see Table 7.3). When BRT commenced, she readily attained criterion on the BRS in both reclined and upright positions (see Figure 7.6). And she maintained her relaxation skills at follow-up. Concurrent with learning to relax in the reclined position, MA's self-rating of tremor during the drinking task mark-

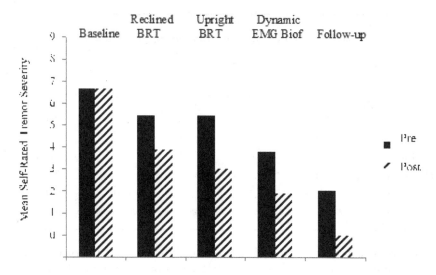

Figure 7.8 Within session mean pre-post training self-rating and post training clinical rating of tremor severity TH while eating with her right hand.

Based on Lundervold, D. A. & Poppen, R. (2004). Biobehavioral intervention for older adults coping with essential tremor. *Applied Psychophysiology and Biofeedback, 29,* 63–74.

edly declined, showing large drops from pre- to post-BRT assessments. Her tremor ratings continued to diminish during the upright BRT and EMG biofeedback phases, as seen in Figure 7.9. And the low SRTS scores were maintained at follow-up. Statistical analysis of these changes showed significant differences between pre- and post-relaxation ratings once treatment began. Each treatment condition was significantly lower than baseline, with upright BRT and dynamic biofeedback resulting in the lowest SRTS scores.

Clinical ratings of tremor were generally lower than self-ratings, but showed the same pattern of change over the treatment conditions. MA's daily home ratings of tremor decreased during the intervention phases, as shown in Table 7.3. Statistical analysis showed her home ratings during treatment to be significantly lower than baseline, though with no differences between treatments phases.

MA received audio feedback based on her biceps EMG during the EMG biofeedback phase due to the observation that biceps EMG increased during ED's biofeedback training phase. Biceps EMG increased with feedback during dynamic movement while extensor EMG initially remained at low levels following upright BRT. As training progressed, extensor EMG markedly increased, prompting a return to reclined BRT in an attempt to reduce muscle tension. Reclined BRT 2 produced a noticeable reduction in EMG levels compared to the pre-training assessment.

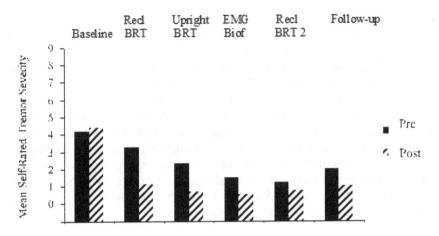

Figure 7.9 Within session mean pre-post self-rating (panel A) and post training clinical rating of tremor severity (Panel B) of MA while drinking with her right hand.

Based on Lundervold, D. A. & Poppen, R. (2004). Biobehavioral intervention for older adults coping with essential tremor. *Applied Psychophysiology and Biofeedback, 29*, 63–74.

Relationships between EMG and other measures were slightly more consistent for MA. After testing for autocorrelation, extensor EMG was analyzed using ANOVA. Extensor EMG was significantly lower at post training assessment indicating a within-session treatment effect. EMG was lowest during upright BRT and dynamic biofeedback conditions with no difference between those conditions. A similar pattern was observed for flexor EMG with flexor EMG lowest during reclined and upright BRT. No other EMG relationships emerged.

Each of the three participants benefited from relaxation training despite the inconsistent relationship been EMG and tremor severity. For each person, performance of functional skills improved following reclined BRT with further improvement in the upright relaxed position. The use of statistical tests allowed a finer-grain analysis of the relative benefit of relaxation and EMG biofeedback to lessen tremor severity. In general, no meaningful difference between upright BRT and dynamic EMG biofeedback emerged. The results of this study also demonstrate the immediate effect of relaxation on ADL performance and also highlight the importance of continued practice to maintain the treatment outcome.

TOURETTE SYNDROME

Tourette Syndrome (TS) is a neurological disorder characterized by repetitive, stereotyped, involuntary movements or vocalizations.[16-18] Common motor tics include eye-blinking, head jerks, or facial movements, while vocal tics can include throat-clearing, tongue-clicking, or verbal utterances. Onset typically occurs in childhood, and boys are three to four times more likely to be affected than girls. Prevalence in the United States has been estimated at six per thousand in children ages 5 to 17. Symptoms may decline with maturation, but many adults continue to struggle with the disorder.

The disruptiveness of symptoms ranges from mild to severe, and may vary over time and circumstances. Frequency of tics may be influenced by events such as environmental stress and emotional arousal, such as anxiety, anger, and excitement. It is difficult to suppress tics, and people who attempt to do so often report a buildup of tension until it bursts forth. Neuroleptic or other psychoactive medication may be helpful for some individuals, but undesirable side-effects are prohibitive for many.

Biobehavioral Treatment of TS

Bergin and colleagues[19] examined the effect of a multicomponent intervention that included reclined BRT, along with PMR, applied relaxation, imaginal exposure, and EMG biofeedback on the severity of tics in children between 7 and 18 years of age. Mean duration of their disorder was 6.7 years, and most were rated in the "mild" range. Tic severity was measured by observer rating scales, while participants also used counters to self-record tic frequency. The relaxation/exposure package was compared to a minimal contact control condition. Participants were randomly assigned to each group. Sixteen participants with TS completed the study. Four children were also diagnosed with attention deficit/hyperactive disorder (ADHD); all of these were assigned to the treatment group.

Six one-hour sessions of the relaxation/exposure intervention were provided to seven youngsters. The trainers used a standard reclining chair to teach relaxation. Participants were instructed to practice relaxation each day and to use applied relaxation in stressful situations or when a tic occurred. Five-minute video recordings of relaxed behavior obtained at baseline, end-of-treatment, and follow-up sessions. The BRS was used to assess relaxed behavior and calculate inter-observer agreement.

Mean baseline BRS score for the two groups did not differ significantly (43% vs. 48%). By the end of training, mean BRS for the treatment group increased to 65 percent relaxed, compared to 41 percent for the controls. Relaxation scores increased slightly for both groups at the 3-month follow-up (73% vs. 45%). Improvement in clinical ratings of tics between groups at post-test approached significance ($p = .07$). Data for self-recorded tic frequency were not reported. Less than half the relaxation group reported compliance with home-practice instructions.

Despite the limitations of small sample size and poor adherence, the results are encouraging. More rigorous training to a higher criterion of 80 to 90 percent relaxed would likely produce better outcomes. Use of extrinsic reinforcers for training and home practice, until the intrinsically reinforcing nature of relaxation occurred, may also increase effectiveness. For small children, a smaller recliner or a beanbag chair can enhance relaxation performance. And the use of single-subject research designs would eliminate the need for a no-treatment control group, allowing more participants to receive training while still demonstrating experimental control.

HUNTINGTON'S DISEASE

Huntington's disease (HD) is a heritable, neurodegenerative disease that affects motor control, cognition, and social behavior. Depression, psychotic disorders, dementia and delirium are common accompaniments.[20] Impaired movement is either *choreiform* (ballistic, irregular involuntary movement), or *dystonic* (sustained contraction of a muscle or muscle group resulting in twisting an appendage into an unusual posture). As in other neurological disorders, symptoms are exacerbated by stress and emotional arousal.[21]

BRT for Choreiform Movements

Fecteau and Boyne[22] evaluated the benefit of BRT with two adults who exhibited choreiform movement and significant cognitive impairment. Both had a positive family history of HD. Participant 1 was a male, age 54, who was stabilized on 325 milligrams of chlorpromazine daily. Participant 2 was a female, age 58, taking no medication at the time of the study.

Participants were randomly assigned to one of two conditions (Baseline or BRT). After completing the first phase, the phases were reversed. Six or seven sessions of BRT were provided. Participant 1 had lost control of voluntary eye blinks and also demonstrated erratic respiration; thus "Eyes" and "Breathing" were removed from scoring on his BRS. During BRT, a blindfold was employed so that he could experience reduced visual stimulation. Baseline sessions were approximately 20 minutes in duration, with the last five minutes used to conduct BRS observation. Heart rate (HR) and frontalis EMG were also measured. Reclined BRT sessions lasted 25 to 30 minutes, the final few minutes of which were spent instructing the participants to observe covert events related to relaxation. A five-minute post-training BRS observation period followed.

Independent *t*-tests were used to compare pooled baseline and training data. Statistically significant increases in BRS scores ($p = .01$) and decreases in HR (p = .05) were observed for BRT as compared to baseline. No EMG differences were found. Participant 1 acquired the eight relaxed behaviors with 100 percent correct performance observed across the last three training sessions. Participant 2 also acquired the relaxed behaviors, with a mean of 90 percent relaxed based on the last three observations. A two-week follow-up indicated the relaxed behaviors were not maintained, though the specific level of performance was not reported.

This study is important in several respects. First, there is no treatment for HD and choreiform movements. Despite significant cognitive impairment, the two participants learned the relaxed behaviors very quickly. Limited maintenance of relaxation skills at a brief follow-up may be due to impaired neurological structures affected by HD.[20] However, no maintenance procedures were implemented. Because of limited options available to patients with HD, these preliminary results encourage further research on the benefits of BRT for persons with HD. It would be useful to include observational measures of choreiform or dystonic movements, and to teach integration of relaxed behaviors into daily routines of patients.

TRAUMATIC BRAIN INJURY

Traumatic brain injury (TBI) is the result of a "blunt or penetrating force to the head" due to rapid acceleration, deceleration, or direct impact, causing alteration in brain function.[23] TBI is a major cause of injury, disability, and mortality among individuals under the age of 45 in the United States.[24] The behavioral sequelae of TBI can be diffuse and involve abrupt and lifelong changes in behavior due to emotional dysregulation, cognitive impairment, and physical disability.[25-27]

The most frequently damaged brain area is the frontal lobes, which affect memory, disinhibition, behavioral and emotional regulation, apathy, judgment, planning, and organization. Impaired cognition severely compromises learning, which leads to behavioral deficits. Task difficulty may elicit maladaptive emotional behavior[26] and set the occasion for escape or avoidance responses.[25,27] Individuals suffering brain injuries incur a variety of changes in behavior, including impulsivity, restlessness, motor impairments, and anxiety.[26,28] These problems suggest that relaxation may be a useful part of a comprehensive treatment plan.

BRT for Psychomotor Difficulties

Zahara[29] demonstrated that persons with TBI could learn relaxation employing BRT. Taylor[30] measured the effects of this training on various psychomotor tasks. Three young men in a residential brain injury treatment facility were referred for relaxation training by their clinical team supervisors, who reported them to be "nervous" or "irritable" and that relaxation would benefit their motor control, social interactions, and general health. Participant 1, 22 years old, had been injured in an automobile accident three years earlier. He manifested both gross and fine motor skill impairments, as in walking and writing. Participant 2, 30 years old, had been injured in an industrial accident more than three years earlier. He displayed impulsivity, restlessness, and social skill deficits. Participant 3, 29 years old, had been injured in a workplace explosion more than one year earlier. His problems included reasoning, memory, and speech impairments.

Training sessions were scheduled three times weekly and lasted approximately 30 minutes, including five minutes of adaptation, 15 minutes of Reclined BRT, and 5 minutes of BRS assessment. Motor skills assessment took place after each session. A multiple-probe-across-participants design was employed, in which baseline measurement sessions were conducted intermittently for two clients while Participant 1 received BRT. When Participant 1 completed acquisition training, BRT was begun for Participant 2. Participant 3 remained in baseline until Participant 2 reached the BRS acquisition criterion.

BRT was trained to an acquisition criterion of 80 percent relaxed on the BRS, followed by six additional proficiency training sessions. An immediate post-training and a three-week follow-up assessment were also conducted. Reliability of BRS scoring was determined by a trained observer in the training room, averaging 90 percent agreement. Frontalis EMG levels and self-report of relaxation also were assessed.

Two psychomotor tasks were conducted with all three participants: a computer game and the placing and turning tests of the Minnesota Rate of Manipulation Test (MRMT). Performances on the computer game and MRMT were measured after alternate BRT sessions. Additional specific performance tasks were assessed for two participants on alternate sessions. Participant 1, who had difficulty writing and signing his name, was tested on a mark-making test while his forearm EMG levels were monitored. Participant 3, who had speaking problems, was tested for duration of breath control while vocalizing vowel sounds.

The participants averaged about 25 percent relaxed behavior during Baseline and showed no improvements over repeated assessment. With BRT, they reached the 80 percent relaxation criterion in four to eight sessions, and maintained or improved this level in subsequent proficiency sessions. Their BRS scores decreased at post-testing and follow-up but did not decline to baseline levels.

Frontalis EMG levels showed no consistent change or relation to BRS scores. This may have been due to scar tissue and other damage related to the participants' head injuries. Self-reports generally reflected an improvement in relaxed feelings during BRT.

No systematic change was observed on the computer games for any participant. Performance on the MRMT improved for Participants 1 and 3, but improvements during Baseline for Participant 3 suggest that this could have been a result of continued practice rather than BRT. Participant 1 showed a large improvement in the mark-making task after BRT, accompanied by a decrease in forearm EMG levels. His therapist reported that he showed much improvement in his everyday writing. Participant 3 showed no change in vowel production duration during baseline but demonstrated a steady increase in duration after relaxation training.

BRT and EMG Biofeedback for Tremor Related to ADL

TBI often results in tremor which impedes performance of activities of daily living, such as eating or buttoning a shirt. Guercio et al.[31] addressed this problem with a 23-year-old man who had sustained a severe closed head injury in an automobile accident. Stephen displayed severe ataxic tremor in arms and hands, requiring significant staff attention during meals, as he could not grasp his utensils or glass firmly enough to prevent spilling. Similarly, he was unable to make coordinated movements needed to smoke a cigarette or place small edibles, such as popcorn, in his mouth.

Stephen's tremor was assessed by recording forearm EMG while he performed two tasks. First, he was asked to use a spoon to transport dry cereal from a bowl to his mouth for approximately two minutes (Eat). The second task was to move a glass of water from one side of a desktop to another, a distance of about two feet (Move). Forearm EMG also was recorded while he sat quietly or relaxed.

A multi-phase intervention program was implemented. During baseline, Stephen was asked to relax as he normally would. A five-minute observation period ensued, during which the BRS was scored and forearm EMG recorded. Then he was asked to perform the Eat and Move tasks. In the BRT phase, Stephen was instructed in and practiced the 10 relaxed postures in the reclined position for 15 to 20 minutes, followed by BRS and EMG recording, and then task performance. In the BRT + biofeedback phase, auditory feedback proportional to forearm muscle tension was provided while he relaxed and also while he performed the eating task. EMG thresholds were set, below which the tone turned off, and these were gradually reduced as tension declined. No biofeedback was given during the move-the-water-glass task. A return-to-baseline phase occurred next, in which Stephen was asked to sit quietly, not necessarily performing the relaxed postures. A second BRT + biofeedback phase was administered. A follow-up session, under baseline conditions, was given six weeks later.

Table 7.4 shows the mean values for each measure across phases. In baseline, when asked to relax on his own, Stephen's BRS scores were very poor. Relaxation improved markedly, to over 90 percent relaxed, when BRT was implemented. Adding EMG biofeedback increased BRS scores somewhat. In the return-to-baseline phase, BRS scores fell, but remained considerably greater than during initial baseline. They improved when BRT + biofeedback was reinstated, and increased to their highest levels at follow-up.

Forearm muscle tension while relaxing was fairly low during baseline, and decreased to less than one microvolt in the BRT phase. Adding auditory feedback paradoxically increased tension levels, averaging 1.65 microvolts (Table 7.4). Perhaps this was due to a floor effect during BRT; it would be difficult to get much below one microvolt. Tension increased during baseline 2 and almost doubled during the second BRT + biofeedback phase. But by follow-up, forearm tension fell to the lowest levels observed.

EMG levels while performing the active tasks of eating (Eat) and moving the water glass (Move), as expected, were much higher than while relaxing (Table 7.4). Activity-related tension decreased noticeably when BRT was implemented, but adding auditory feedback while performing the Eat task

Table 7.4
Mean value across experimental phases for each dependent measure for Stephen.

	Phase					
Measure	Baseline	BRT	BRT + BIO	Baseline 2	BRT+BIO2	FU
BRS % Relaxed	11.2	91.0	85.6	60.0	84.4	94.0
EMG: Relax microvolts	2.17	0.98	1.65	5.51	9.87	0.61
EMG Eat microvolts	67.5	33.5	36.9	51.5	35.2	38.0
EMG Move microvolts	41.0	32.9	34.9	56.2	39.1	31.0

Based on Guercio, J., Chittum, W.R., & McMorrow, M.J. (1997). Self-management in the treatment of ataxia: A case study in reducing ataxic tremor through relaxation and biofeedback. *Brain Injury*, *11*(5), 353–362.

had little discernible effect. Tension increased during return-to-baseline but declined during the subsequent BRT + biofeedback phase, and remained at low levels during follow-up.

In summary, forearm muscle tension decreased when BRT was implemented, both while engaging in relaxation and afterwards, while performing active tasks associated with daily living. EMG biofeedback did not enhance the effects of relaxation and may have resulted in slight decrements in performance. Decreases in muscle tension may be related to reducing tremor and improving ability to perform everyday activities. Clinical staff reported that Stephen needed much less assistance for eating and drinking after participating in the study.

BRT and EMG Biofeedback for Tremor Related to Functional Communication

Individuals suffering TBI frequently have impaired communication skills due to injury of specific brain areas involved in speech and language. Impaired motor responses may also impede use of augmentative communication devices. Guercio[32] and colleagues (2001) used BRT combined with EMG biofeedback to reduce ataxic tremor, resulting in improved performance on a communication device.

Hugh, a 21-year-old male, had sustained brain injury as well as a broken right arm and numerous internal lacerations in an automobile-train collision five years prior. He later developed hydrocephalus and a shunt was put in place to address this. At the time of the study, hemiparesis was noted on Hugh's right side and he experienced severe ataxic tremor in his left arm during purposeful movement (kinetic tremor). He utilized a wheelchair but required maximal assistance from staff for locomotion. Hugh had severe dysarthria and very rudimentary speech; he could express some basic needs with yes/no responses or by pointing, but used a spell board for more extensive verbal interactions.

Hugh's performance was recorded on three measures. Relaxation was measured by the BRS. Muscle tension in the flexors and extensors of his left forearm, while performing a spelling task, was measured by an EMG device. The spelling task consisted three trials in which he was asked to spell various simple phrases (e.g., "My name is Hugh"). Tremor severity during the spelling task was rated by the trainer using the Clinical Rating of Tremor Severity scale (CRTS).[13] Reliability of observation on both the BRS and the CRTS was over 90 percent.

Treatment consisted of a baseline phase, during which Hugh was seated in a reclining chair and asked to relax on his own for ten minutes, followed by the spelling task. In the BRT phase, Hugh was instructed in the relaxed

Table 7.5
Mean values across experimental phases for each dependent measure for Hugh

Measure	Phase					
	Baseline	BRT	BIOF1	BIOF2	BIOF3	Follow Up
BRS % Relaxed	15.3	74.3	77.0	89.5	91.0	90.0
EMG microvolts	68.1	57.7	44.9	39.8	36.2	40.9
CRTS	7.0	3.9	3.0	2.8	3.0	3.0

Based on Guercio, J.M., Ferguson, K.E., & McMorrow, M.J. (2001). Increasing functional communication abilities through relaxation training and neuromuscular feedback. *Brain Injury*, 15 (12), 1073–1082.

postures, followed by a five-minute BRS scoring period, and then the spelling task. In the BRT + biofeedback phase, Hugh first relaxed, the BRS was scored, then during the spelling task he was provided with an auditory signal if his forearm EMG exceeded a certain threshold value. Decreasing tension turned the signal off. The threshold level was decreased in successive phases to the mean of the preceding phase. A follow-up session, two years after completion of training, consisted of one session of relaxation with no instruction, and spelling task performance with no biofeedback.

Table 7.5 displays Hugh's performance across the phases of the study. Mean values of each dependent measure are given. BRS scores were very low in Baseline, averaging only 15 percent relaxed. They improved immediately when BRT was implemented and continued to increase across phases when forearm EMG biofeedback was given for the spelling task. At follow-up, a BRS score of 90 percent relaxed was obtained.

Muscle tension, measured by forearm EMG, decreased as relaxation performance improved. This suggests that relaxation carried over from the recliner to performance on the spelling task. The mean EMG level for each phase served as the threshold for the successive phase. It is likely that relaxation and EMG biofeedback had a synergistic relationship, enabling lower and lower threshold values to be set. Hugh's low EMG level was maintained at follow-up.

Tremor ratings while Hugh performed the spelling task were consistent with the other measures. Baseline ratings averaged 7.0, in the "severe" tremor range. This decreased almost by half in the BRT phase, declined further to the "mild" range with biofeedback training, and was maintained at follow-up. The authors noted that Hugh was able to maintain his relaxation skills, decreased forearm EMG values, and mild tremor levels, at a two-year follow-up even though facilities at his residence were not favorable for regular practice.

CONCLUSION

Behavioral relaxation training has been repeatedly demonstrated to be of benefit to individuals with diverse neurological disorders, and has allowed them to more effectively manage impaired movement and improve their performance of activities of daily living. The research in this section has also shown that that there is not always complete correspondence between biological response systems, overt behavior, and self-reported performance. Consequently, multimodal-multibehavior measurement systems are needed to adequately assess the effects of relaxation, especially among individuals with neurological disorders and diseases. While the use of biomonitoring is of value in establishing interrelationships among response modalities, in many cases the addition of biofeedback interventions provides no more benefit than BRT. Because of the costs and additional training needed to use biofeedback, BRT remains the first best step in addressing the diverse needs of individuals with neurological disorders.

REFERENCES

[1]Louis, E. D., Ottman, R., & Hauser, W. A. (1998). How common is the most common adult movement disorder? Estimates of the prevalence of essential tremor throughout the world. *Movement Disorders, 13*(1), 5–10. https://doi.org/10.1002/mds.870130105

[2]Louis, E. D. (2009). Essential tremors: a family of neurodegenerative disorders? *Archives of Neurology, 66*(10), 1202–1208. https://doi.org/10.1001/archneurol.2009.217

[3]Elble, R. J. (2017). Tremor. In B. Tousi, & J. Cummings, (Eds.) *Neuro-Geriatrics. A clinical manual* (pp 311–326). New York: Springer International Publishing.

[4]Louis, E. D., Barnes, L., Albert, S. M., Cote, L., Schneier, F. R., Pullman, S. L., & Yu, Q. (2001). Correlates of functional disability in essential tremor. *Movement Disorders, 16*(5), 914–920. https://doi.org/10.1002/mds.1184

[5]Chandrana, V., & Kumar, P. (2013). Quality of life and its determinants in essential tremor. *Parkinsonism & Related Disorders, 19*(1), 62–65. https://doi.org/10.1016/j.parkreldis.2012.06.011

[6]Schneier, F. R., Barnes, L. F., Albert, S. M., & Louis, E. D. (2001). Characteristics of social phobia among persons with essential tremor. *Journal of Clinical Psychiatry, 62*(5), 367–372. https://doi.org/10.4088/JCP.v62n0511

[7]Lundervold, D. A., Ament, P. A., & Holt, P. (2013). Social anxiety, tremor severity, and tremor disability: A search for clinically relevant measures. *Psychiatry Journal, Volume 2013, Article ID 257459, 5 pages.* http://dx.doi.org/10.1155/2013/257459

[8]Mattick, R. P., & Clarke, J. C. (1998). Development and validation of measures of social phobia scrutiny fear and social interaction anxiety. *Behavior Research and Therapy, 36*(4), 455–470. https://doi.org/10.1016/S0005-7967(97)10031-6

[9]Louis, E. D., Rohl, B., & Rice, C. (2015). Defining the treatment gap: What essential tremor patients want that they are not getting. *Tremor Other Hyperkinet Mov (NY). 2015; 5: 331.*

[10]Chung, W., Poppen, R., & Lundervold, D. A. (1995). Behavioral relaxation training for tremor disorders in older adults. *Biofeedback and Self-Regulation, 20,* 123–135. https://doi.org/10.1007/BF01720969

[11]Fahn, S., Elton, R. L., & UPDRS program members. Unified Parkinson's Disease Rating Scale. (1987). In S. Fahn, C.D. Marsden, M. Goldstein, & D. B. Calne, (Eds.), *Recent developments in Parkinson's disease, 2,* (pp. 153–163). Florham Park, NJ: Macmillan Healthcare Information.

[12]Lundervold, D. A., Belwood, M. F., Craney, J. C., & Poppen, R. (1999). Reduction of tremor severity and disability following behavioral relaxation training. *Journal of Behavior Therapy and Experimental Psychiatry, 30,* 119–135. https://doi.org/10.1016/S0005-7916(99) 00015-4

[13]Bain, P. G. (1993). A combined clinical and neurophysiological approach to the study of patients with essential tremor. *Journal of Neurology, Neurosurgery, and Psychiatry, 56,* 839–844. https://doi.org/10.1136/jnnp.56.8.839

[14]Lundervold, D. A., & Poppen, R. (2004). Relaxation and biofeedback training for tremor-related disability. *Applied Psychophysiology and Biofeedback, 29*(1):63–73. https://doi.org/10.1023/B:APBI.0000017864.06525.eb

[15]Elble, R. J., & Koller, W. C. (1990). *Tremor*. Baltimore: Johns Hopkins University Press.

[16]American Psychiatric Association. (2013). *Diagnostic and Statistical Manual of Mental Disorders., 5th edition*. Washington, DC: American Psychiatric Association Press.

[17]Tourette Association of America. Retrieved June 27, 2019 from https://tourette.org/about-tourette/overview/faqs/.

[18]National Institute of Neurological and Communication Disorders. Retrieved June 27, 2019 from https://www.ninds.nih.gov/Disorders/Patient-Caregiver-Education.

[19]Bergin, A., Waranch, H. R., Brown, J., Carson, K., & Singer, H. S. (1998). Relaxation therapy in Tourette syndrome: A pilot study. *Pediatric Neurology, 18*(2), 136–142. https://doi.org/10.1016/S0887-8994(97)00200-2

[20]Rosenblatt, A. (2007). Neuropsychiatry of Huntington's disease. *Dialogues in Clinical Neuroscience, 9*(2), 191–197. Retrieved January 20, 2019 from https://www.ncbi.nlm.nih.gov/pmc/articles/PMC3181855/

[21]Esch, T., Stefan, G. B., Fricchione, G. L., & Benson, H. (2001). The role of stress in neurodegenerative diseases and mental disorders. *Neuroendocrinology Letters, 23*,199–208.

[22]Fecteau, G. W., & Boyne, J. (1987). Behavioral relaxation training with Huntington's disease patients: A pilot study. *Psychological Reports, 81*, 151–157. https://doi.org/10.2466/pr0.1987.61.1.151

[23]Zollman, F. S. (2011). *Manual of Traumatic Brain Injury Management*. New York: Demos Medical Publishing.

[24]Bruns, J., & Hauser, W. A. (2003). The epidemiology of traumatic brain injury: A review. *Epilepsia, 44*(10), 2–10.38. https://doi.org/10.1046/j.1528-1157.44.s10.3.x

[25]Ducharme, J. M. (2000). Treatment of maladaptive behavior in acquired brain injury: remedial approaches in post acute settings. *Clinical Psychology Review, 20*(3), 40–426.47. https://doi.org/10.1016/S0272-7358(98)00102-0

[26]Hiott, D. W., & Labbate, L. (2002). Anxiety disorders associated with traumatic brain injuries. *NeuroRehabilitation, 17*, 345–355.

[27]Zahara, D. J., & Cuvo, A. J. (1984). Behavioral applications to the rehabilitation of traumatically head injured persons. *Clinical Psychology Review, 4*(4), 477–491. https://doi.org/10.1016/0272-7358(84)90022-9

[28]Yody, B. B., Schaub, C., Conway, J., Peters, S., Strauss, D., & Helsinger, S. (2000). Applied behavior management and acquired brain injury: approaches and assessment. *Journal of Head Trauma Rehabilitation, 15*(4), 1041–1060. https://doi.org/10.1097/00001199-200008000-00006

[29]Zahara, D. (1983). *Behavioral relaxation training with traumatically head-injured adults*. Unpublished master's thesis, Southern Illinois University at Carbondale.

[30]Taylor, S. L. (1983). *Behavioral relaxation training and assessment with traumatically brain-injured adults: Effects on motor performance*. Unpublished master's thesis, Southern Illinois University at Carbondale.

[31]Guercio, J., Chittum, W. R., & McMorrow, M. J. (1997). Self-management in the treatment of ataxia: A case study in reducing ataxic tremor through relaxation and biofeedback. *Brain Injury, 11*(5), 353–362. https://doi.org/10.1080/026990597123511

[32]Guercio, J. M., Ferguson, K. E., & McMorrow, M. J. (2001). Increasing functional communication abilities through relaxation training and neuromuscular feedback. *Brain Injury, 15*(12), 1073–1082. https://doi.org/10.1080/02699050110065673

Supplement
Behavior Analyst Certification Board 5th Edition Task List

A. Philosophical Underpinnings
A-1   Identify the goals of behavior analysis as a science (i.e., description, prediction, control).
A-2   Explain the philosophical assumptions underlying the science of behavior analysis (e.g., selectionism, determinism, empiricism, parsimony, pragmatism).
A-3   Describe and explain behavior from the perspective of radical behaviorism.
A-4   Distinguish among behaviorism, the experimental analysis of behavior, applied behavior analysis, and professional practice guided by the science of behavior analysis.
A-5   Describe and define the dimensions of applied behavior analysis (Baer, Wolf, & Risley, (1968).

B. Concepts and Principles
B-3   Define and provide examples of respondent and operant conditioning.
B-4   Define and provide examples of positive and negative reinforcement contingencies.
B-5   Define and provide examples of schedules of reinforcement.

C. Measurement, Data Display, and Interpretation
C-1   Establish operational definitions of behavior.
C-2   Distinguish among direct, indirect, and product measures of behavior.
C-3   Measure occurrence (e.g., frequency, rate, percentage).
C-5   Measure form and strength of behavior (e.g., topography, magnitude).
C-6   Measure trials to criterion.
C-7   Design and implement sampling procedures (i.e., interval recording, time sampling).
C-8   Evaluate the validity and reliability of measurement procedures.
C-9   Select a measurement system to obtain representative data given the dimensions of behavior and the logistics of observing and recording.
C-10   Graph data to communicate relevant quantitative relations (e.g., equal-interval graphs, bar graphs, cumulative records).
C-11   Interpret graphed data.

D. Experimental Design
D-1 Distinguish between dependent and independent variables.
D-5 Use single-subject experimental designs (e.g., reversal, multiple baseline, multielement, changing criterion).

G. Behavior-Change Procedures
G-1 Use positive and negative reinforcement procedures to strengthen behavior.
G-5 Use modeling and imitation training.
G-6 Use instructions and rules.
G-9 Use discrete-trial, free-operant, and naturalistic teaching arrangements.
G-14 Use reinforcement procedures to weaken behavior (e.g., DRA, FCT, DRO, DRL, NCR).
G-20 Use self-management strategies.

H. Selecting and Implementing Interventions
H-1 State intervention goals in observable and measurable terms.
H-4 When a target behavior is to be decreased, select an acceptable alternative behavior to be established or increased.
H-6 Monitor client progress and treatment integrity.
H-7 Make data-based decisions about the effectiveness of the intervention and the need for treatment revision.
H-9 Collaborate with others who support and/or provide services to clients.

Chapter 8

Where Do We Go From Here?

BRT and the BRS have been established as evidence-based relaxation training and assessment procedures. However, questions about relaxation in general, and about BRT and the BRS remain. Here we present several questions that were raised throughout the book that fall under two categories: (a) the basic nature of relaxation; and, (b) its clinical significance. In most cases, relaxation is employed to reach clinical goals, though not always.[1]

BASIC RESEARCH QUESTIONS

The fundamental issue remains the same: What is the nature of relaxation? Like the parable of the blind men and the elephant, various investigators have asserted that relaxation is, among other things, parasympathetic dominance, motoneuron quiescence, or a cognitive state of calm. Ignoring the problems of assessment for the moment, each of these may be part of the picture but none is the whole "elephant." Perhaps a better metaphor would be the chameleon, reflecting the idea that relaxation is different things in different situations for different people. As presented in this book, relaxation is a response class comprised of four modalities: motor, verbal, visceral, and observational. The elements of the relaxation response class differ depending on environmental and individual variables. By changing the focus from a search for an elusive "state" to a functional analysis of behavior, the chameleon can be better described.

What Are the Common and Specific Effects of Different Training Methods?

A major question concerns what often are termed "placebo" effects. These may be more accurately called effects of the "common elements" of relaxation training procedures. As described in Chapter 1, there are many training procedures. The distinction is that common elements are not inert (as implied by the term "placebo") but rather are active variables influencing behavior. Because they are an inextricable part of most training procedures, it is difficult to control for them by omission; that is, the appropriate research design is not a comparison of the presence versus the absence of these variables (as in "double-blind" medical research) but rather is a comparison of qualities and levels of these elements.

Common treatment elements involve certain antecedents, behaviors and consequences. The antecedents typically include "rules" or the rationale for training, an authority with special knowledge, an unwanted condition for which relaxation is said to be helpful, and a quiet place for training and practice. The behaviors include routine cessation of ongoing activities, observation of a repetitive low-intensity event, a comfortable posture, and self-report of progress. The consequences include social approval for success, social support for failure, and the promise of alleviation of the unwanted condition.

In this context the questions are many. What does BRT (or any relaxation procedure) add to this general format? What are the effects of performing specific relaxation actions and observing oneself doing so, as opposed to engaging in some other motor and observational behavior? Are differential effects obtained when engaging in different relaxation behaviors that are based on other theories/procedures of relaxation? Research comparing various relaxation methods is beginning to address these questions, but cannot be done in blanket terms of "better" or "worse." Effects in all behavior modalities should be considered, though unfortunately this has seldom been done. Efforts to detect changes within and across modalities other than the targeted ones should be increased. For example, within the motor domain, Poppen and Maurer[2] found that EMG biofeedback for reducing tension produces relaxed postures and that producing relaxed postures reduces EMG levels. But what are the effects of motor training on verbal, visceral, and observational behaviors? Similarly, verbally guided observational procedures, such as autogenic training or meditation, may produce verbal and observational changes, but do they also have the visceral or motor effects that are hypothesized?

Which Dependent Measures?

Efforts to determine relaxation effects within and across behavior modalities raise questions about what measures to use, as well as questions about their reliability and validity. Research establishing the reliability and validity of the BRS was described in Chapter 3, with applications described through the remainder of the book. The BRS is a measure of motor behavior, and measures of relaxation in other modalities are needed. Assessment of the verbal and observational domain may be aided by use of the STAR, discussed earlier. EMG activity is a widely accepted motor measure of relaxation, but there are unanswered questions even with this. For example, multisite EMG recording rarely is employed, and little is known about patterns or generalization of muscle activity. For example, the effect of BRT on visceral behavior remains unexamined.

While self-report questionnaires of relaxation have been developed,[3,4] the construct validity of these measures has not been replicated by independent investigators.[5] As a valid measure of the motor effects of relaxation and a direct observation measure of relaxed behavior, the BRS stands as an evidence-based metric that should be used to compare other relaxation measurement devices such as clinical and self-report rating scales.[6]

Visceral and observational behaviors are notoriously difficult to measure, as discussed in Chapter 2. Yet these modalities play an important role in many problematic behaviors and in relaxation. Difficulty in measurement poses a challenge to be taken up by researchers rather than avoided.

QUESTIONS OF CLINICAL SIGNIFICANCE

Beyond the questions concerning which modalities of behavior are affected by training, is the matter of how these are related to treatment outcome. The relationship between proficiency in relaxation and treatment outcome is a valid research question.

Process Measures and Treatment Outcome

What we are proposing is a multibehavior-multimethod approach to the behavioral assessment of the effects of relaxation. All members of the relaxation response class need to be included in the equation.

Wittrock, Blanchard, and McCoy[7] present a model examining the relationship between process and outcome measures that may be employed and further developed. Of interest was how self-efficacy (a verbal rating of the extent to which one can learn/perform a skill), outcome expectations (verbal rating of the extent to which one's actions will influence an outcome), and level of skill acquisition are related to symptom reduction. Participants who had higher expectations were more successful in symptom reduction (blood pressure readings). With respect to skill acquisition, research on hypertension has shown that individuals who report "deeper relaxation" also have greater symptom reduction. The limitation of this research is that direct measurement of relaxed behavior was not obtained and the training criterion varied across participants. Wittrock et al. also demonstrated that fluency in relaxation skills resulted in more substantial decreases in blood pressure. Participants' verbal report of the extent ("depth") of relaxation also predicted treatment success. Lundervold and Poppen[8] demonstrated that meeting relaxation training criteria as measured by the BRS was significantly correlated with reduced EMG and self- and clinician-rated symptom reduction.

In cases in which there is a hypothesized mechanism of action in a specific behavior domain, such as muscle tension as related to headache or back pain, it is particularly important to assess changes in that domain. This can lend support to the formulation or can suggest that another mechanism needs to be investigated. Measures need to be obtained not only in the clinical setting but also in the participant's home environment.

The behavior analytic treatment strategy assumes that the trainer is not simply providing "doses" of relaxation in the clinic, but rather is teaching skills that must be transferred to the participant's everyday environment. This is a testable assumption. Improvements in electronic technology and miniaturization make portable EMG and visceral measures more available to clinical researchers, although these still are beyond the reach of practicing clinicians. The BRS, Upright Behavioral Relaxation Scale (UBRS), informant, and self-report measure of relaxation (See Appendices A-C, E, G, H) provide non-electronic measures, though the reliability and construct validity of these BRS-based indirect measures of relaxed behavior is needed.

BRT, like progressive relaxation and EMG biofeedback, is assumed to target changes in motor behavior (muscle tension) that is measurable by the BRS. Changes in the BRS (and EMG levels) in the training and home environment can be related to changes in symptoms, allowing testing of this treatment hypothesis.[8] The case studies described in Chapters 5 through 7 begin to address this important clinical and research question. As described Chapter 6, caregivers and independent observers can be trained to score an approximation to or the actual BRS.

Clinical Effects of BRT

Numerous case studies have been presented throughout the book demonstrating the benefit of BRT, but more controlled treatment outcome studies are needed. Many stress and pain disorders are assumed to have muscle tension or muscle asymmetry as a major component. For example, tension headache, fibromyalgia, and lower back pain lend themselves to treatment with BRT. Because of the ease of training, and the rapid learning of the relaxed behaviors by most individuals, BRT is proposed as a more efficient alternative to other motor methods, such as progressive relaxation or EMG biofeedback. Research is needed to empirically demonstrate the efficiency benefit. Or, in certain instances, BRT may be combined with other methods to form a more potent package, but, yet again, research is needed to determine if such a benefit exists or outweighs the extra time and effort required.

In addition to motor disorders, BRT can be applied with disorders in other domains. It can be combined beneficially with visceral procedures, such as thermal biofeedback or diaphragmatic breathing, for intervention with viscerally related problems such as asthma, panic attack, hypertension, and migraine. BRT may act in a synergistic fashion with observational procedures, such as guided imagery, for intervention with the observational component of disorders such as chronic pain or anxiety. Similarly, BRT may be augmented with verbal techniques such as autogenic training for problems in the verbal domain. All the suggested combinations of BRT with other methods, as described in an earlier section, still await empirical validation.

Chapters 5 and 6 described the application of BRT to arousal-related disorders. The evidence indicates BRT is especially useful for persons with intellectual disabilities, with some suggestion that it is equally effective with persons with autism spectrum disorder. Learning relaxation skills provides such individuals an important means to manage their behavior independently, or with minimal external assistance. In this regard, BRT is an especially valuable procedure that teaches replacement behaviors that serve the same response function as maladaptive behavior. More research is needed to demonstrate that persons with intellectual disabilities, autism spectrum disorders, or traumatic brain injury, can learn relaxation and that it has a beneficial effect on their daily lives. The work of Guercio[9] hints that such is the case. More studies comparing and combining methods are needed for persons in these populations.

Questions about treatment efficiency suggest a different sort of research design from that usually employed. A common procedure has been to give a fixed number of treatment sessions and assess outcome in terms of average improvement on various measures among individuals in treatment and control groups. An alternative design is to measure the number of trials required to achieve a pre-set improvement criterion for proficiency in relaxed behaviors and symptom change. This can be accomplished in both single-subject and group research design. This method more closely approximates clinical practice in which treatment continues until some level of satisfaction is reached.[10] The question of efficiency of acquisition of skills and treatment effect is especially important as behavioral health care providers become more and more integrated into primary and tertiary care medical settings.[11]

THE CLINICIAN AS RESEARCHER

This book presents many examples of how a treatment provider can contribute to the scientific literature that reinforces the evidence-based foundations of behavior analytic-based intervention. This comes at some cost in time and effort to both the clinician and the participant, but we and others maintain that the payoff to the participants and to our knowledge base is well worth it.[12] Some methodological requirements are sketched below.

First, informed consent must be obtained which is a necessary part of providing care. The consent form can easily be modified to include a description of how a participant's data may be shared with other professionals and students for educational purposes. This section can include a check-off box for the participant to indicate yes or no relative to use of their data. As part of the description, participants (or agents responsible for their care) are informed that they will remain anonymous in any sharing of information in educational settings such as classrooms, conferences, or the publication of manuscripts. Participants are also informed that refusing to share their data will result in no denial of services or any other penalty. Individuals who are referred or recruited because the clinician has expertise in an area or interest in their condition are typically eager to participate.

Function-based assessment is crucial. Simply using self-reports of subjective states is inadequate. Depending on context, function-based assessment may include indirect measures such as a function-based behavior interview[13-15] and direct assessment of challenging behavior, and, of course, relaxation. Multimodal and process measures, as noted above, are much-needed contributions. Outcome assessment provides assurance to both clinician and participant of treatment effectiveness. Or in negative instances, it suggests possible alternative interventions. Adequate assessment requires baseline and follow-up periods, and ideally should include measurements in environments outside the treatment setting.

Single-subject research designs[16,17] are very useful when working with individuals or small numbers of participants. Repeated measurement, necessary for such research, keeps both clinician and participant focused on the task at hand. Because in most cases we are teaching skills to be maintained and generalized, reversal designs are contraindicated. Multiple baseline across treatment components, settings, or individuals often fill the bill. When the statistical assumptions about the data are met, parametric statistical analysis allows more certain conclusions about treatment phases than mere descriptive analysis, and is often the coin of the realm with respect to interpreting treatment effects. New approaches to synthesis of data obtained from single-subject research designs, such as baseline corrected TAU[18-20] and corrected percentage of data above the median (PEM)[17,20] provide an easy means to determine a statistical effect size[18,19] or a reliable estimate of a change from baseline.[17] We are sure that innovations in single-subject research design and data analytic methods will evolve as relaxation research expands.

CONCLUSION

The evidence for the efficacy and efficiency of BRT has grown since its origins thirty years ago, and the future of BRT remains bright. Similarly, the BRS has opened the door to issues in the assessment of relaxation. We hope that this book will serve as an antecedent for clinicians and researchers from a variety of theoretical orientations to join in the investigation and use of BRT and related measures in practice.

Beyond the specific issues of BRT and the BRS as means of training and assessing relaxation, it is hoped that the four-modality response system theory presented here will generate a new look at complex behavior in general, and relaxation specifically. Presenting the various relaxation methods and theories from a behavior analytic viewpoint allows an empirical basis for comparison and evaluation research. Much hard work remains to be done before we can kick back and relax.

REFERENCES

[1]Scheufele, P. M. (2000). Effects of progressive relaxation and classical music on measurements of attention, relaxation and stress responses. *Journal of Behavioral Medicine, 23*, 207–228. https://doi.org/10.1023/A:1005542121935

[2]Poppen, R., & Maurer, J. (1982). Electromyographic analysis of relaxed postures. *Biofeedback and Self-Regulation, 7*, 491–498. https://doi.org/10.1007/BF00998889

[3]Crist, D. A., Rickard, H. C., Prentice-Dunn, S., & Barker, H. R. (1989). The Relaxation Inventory: Self-report scales of relaxation training effects. *Journal of Personality Assessment, 53*, 716–726. https://doi.org/10.1207/s15327752jpa5304_8

[4]Smith, J. C. (2001). *Advances in ABC relaxation: Applications and inventories.* NY: Springer.

[5]Hites, L. S., & Lundervold, D. A. (2013). Relation between direct observation of relaxation and self-reported mindfulness and relaxation states. *International Journal of Behavioral Consultation and Therapy, 7*(4), 6–7. https://doi.org/10.1037/h0100958

[6]Lundervold, D. A., Kopp, R, Garcia, A., Fontanette, T., & Ament, P. A. (2014). *States of arousal and relaxation (STAR) questionnaire measures mindfulness.* Association for Psychological Science, San Francisco, CA.

[7]Wittrock, D. A., Blanchard, E. B., & McCoy, G. C. (1988). Three studies on the relation of process to outcome in the treatment of essential hypertension with relaxation and thermal biofeedback. *Behavior Research and Therapy, 26*(1), 53–66. http://dx.doi.org/10.1016/0005-7967(88)90033-2

[8]Lundervold, D. A., & Poppen, R. (2004). Biobehavioral intervention for older adults coping with essential tremor. *Applied Psychophysiology and Biofeedback, 29*(1):63–73. https://doi.org/10.1023/B:APBI.0000017864.06525.eb

[9]Guercio, J. M. (2018). *Use of Behavioral Relaxation Training to manage stress-related self-injurious, aggressive and property destruction of an adult with autism spectrum disorder and intellectual disability.* Unpublished manuscript.

[10]Poppen, R. (1983). Clinical practice and biofeedback research: Are the machines necessary? *The Behavior Therapist, 6,* 145–148.

[11]Lundervold, D. A., Holt, P., Beasley, B. W., & Pahwa, R. (2019). *A perfect storm of opportunity: Integrated health care, evidence-based practice, and single case research design.* Unpublished manuscript.

[12]Lister, K. E., & Moody, S. J. (2017). Cutting the profession's Gordian Knot: A call for evidence-based practice in counseling. *Journal of Counselor Leadership and Advocacy, 4*(2), 137–146. https://doi.org/10.1080/2326716X.2017.1322930

[13]Kanfer, F. H., & Saslow, G. (1965). Behavioral analysis. An alternative to diagnostic classification. *Archives of General Psychiatry, 12*(6) 529–538. https://doi.org/10.1001/archpsyc.1965.01720360001001

[14]Haynes, S. N., & O'Brien, W. H. (2000). *Applied clinical psychology. Principles and practice of behavioral assessment.* Kluwer Academic/Plenum Publishers: NY.

[15]O'Neill, R. E., Horner, R. H., Albin, R. W., Sprague, J. R., Storey, K., & Newton, J. S. (1997). *Functional assessment and program development for problem behavior.* Pacific Grove, CA: Brooks/Cole Publishing.

[16]Lundervold, D. A., & Belwood, M. F. (2000). The best kept secret in counseling: Single case (N=1) experimental designs. *Journal of Counseling and Development, 78*(1), 92–102. https://doi.org/10.1002/j.1556-6676.2000.tb02565.x

[17]Morley, S. (2017). *Single case methods in clinical psychology.* Taylor & Francis Group: London.

[18]Tarlow, K. R. (2016). An improved rank correlation effect size statistic for single-case designs: Baseline corrected Tau. *Behavior Modification, 41*(4), 427–467. https://doi.org/10.1177/0145445516676750

[19]*Baseline corrected tau/Kevin Tarlow.* Retrieved November 13, 2019 from http://ktarlow.com/stats/tau/.

[20]Hammond, K., & Lundervold, D.A. (2019). *Examination of TAU, baseline corrected TAU, and PEM using single subject research design data.* Mid-American Association for Behavior Analysis, Omaha, NE.

Supplement
Behavior Analyst Certification Board 5ᵗʰ Edition Task List

A. Philosophical Underpinnings
A-1 Identify the goals of behavior analysis as a science (i.e., description, prediction, control).
A-2 Explain the philosophical assumptions underlying the science of behavior analysis (e.g., selectionism, determinism, empiricism, parsimony, pragmatism).
A-3 Describe and explain behavior from the perspective of radical behaviorism.
A-4 Distinguish among behaviorism, the experimental analysis of behavior, applied behavior analysis, and the practice guided by the science of behavior analysis.
A-5 Describe and define the dimensions of applied behavior analysis (Baer, Wolf, & Risley, 1968).

B. Concepts and Principles
B-1 Define and provide examples of behavior, response, and response class.

C. Measurement, Data Display, and Interpretation
C-1 Establish operational definitions of behavior.
C-2 Distinguish among direct, indirect and product measures of behavior.
C-3 Measure the occurrence (e.g., frequency, rate, percentage).
C-5 Measure the form and strength of the behavior (e.g., topography, magnitude).
C-6 Measure trials to criterion.

D. Experimental Design
D-1 Distinguish between dependent and independent variables.
D-5 Use single-subject research designs (e.g., reversal, multiple baseline, multielement, changing criterion).
D-6 Discuss the rationale for conducting comparative, component, and parametric analyses.

E. Ethics
E-1 Responsible conduct of behavior analysts.
E-2 Behavior analysts' responsibility to clients.
E-3 Behavior analysts and behavior-change program.

E-6   Behavior analysts' ethical responsibility to the profession of behavior analysis.
E-9   Behavior analysts and research.

F. Behavior Assessment
F-6   Describe common functions of problem behavior.
F-6   Conduct descriptive assessment of problem behavior.

Appendices

Appendix A
Tension Self-Rating Scale

Tension Self-Rating Scale and Home Practice Recording Form

Name _____ Phase: Reclined   Upright   FU

Instructions: Record the date. Immediately before and immediately after relaxing rate your level of tension using the scale below. The record what behaviors were difficult to relax.

Rating Scale

7=Feeling extremely tense throughout my body
6=Feeling generally tense throughout my body
5=Feeling some tension in some areas of my body
4=Feeling relaxed as in my normal resting state
3=Feeling more relaxed than in my normal resting state
2=Feeling deeply and completely relaxed throughout my body
1=Feeling more deeply and completely relaxed than I ever have

Date	Tension before	Tension after	Duration	difficult to relax?

Appendix B
States of Arousal and Relaxation Scale

Name _____   Condition: Baseline   RBRT   UBRT   FU

Instructions: Please record what you noticed, felt or experienced as you were relaxing. Circle a number that best describes you.

1. I felt refreshed.

1	2	3	4	5	6	7
much less than before	less than before	slightly less than before	normal; no different	slightly more than before	more thsn before	much more than before

2. I felt enlivened.

1	2	3	4	5	6	7
much less than before	less than before	slightly less than before	normal; no different	slightly more than before	more thsn before	much more than before

3. I felt reinvigorated.

1	2	3	4	5	6	7
much less than before	less than before	slightly less than before	normal; no different	slightly more than before	more thsn before	much more than before

4. I felt revived.

1	2	3	4	5	6	7
much less than before	less than before	slightly less than before	normal; no different	slightly more than before	more thsn before	much more than before

5. I felt detached from my surroundings.

1	2	3	4	5	6	7
much less than before	less than before	slightly less than before	normal; no different	slightly more than before	more thsn before	much more than before

6. I felt disconnected from my body and mind.

1	2	3	4	5	6	7
much less than before	less than before	slightly less than before	normal; no different	slightly more than before	more thsn before	much more than before

7. I felt separate from my body, as if I were floating.

1	2	3	4	5	6	7
much less than before	less than before	slightly less than before	normal; no different	slightly more than before	more thsn before	much more than before

8. I felt cut loose, adrift from my mind and body.

1	2	3	4	5	6	7
much less than before	less than before	slightly less than before	normal; no different	slightly more than before	more thsn before	much more than before

9. My mind was hushed.

1	2	3	4	5	6	7
much less than before	less than before	slightly less than before	normal; no different	slightly more than before	more thsn before	much more than before

10. My thoughts were muted and quiet.

1	2	3	4	5	6	7
much less than before	less than before	slightly less than before	normal; no different	slightly more than before	more thsn before	much more than before

11. Distracting thoughts and images were subdued and still.

1	2	3	4	5	6	7
much less than before	less than before	slightly less than before	normal; no different	slightly more than before	more thsn before	much more than before

12. My mind was silent.

1	2	3	4	5	6	7
much less than before	less than before	slightly less than before	normal; no different	slightly more than before	more thsn before	much more than before

13. I am aware of sensations or feelings in my body.

1	2	3	4	5	6	7
much less than before	less than before	slightly less than before	normal; no different	slightly more than before	more thsn before	much more than before

14.   I notice physical sensations of my body.

1	2	3	4	5	6	7
much less than before	less than before	slightly less than before	normal; no different	slightly more than before	more thsn before	much more than before

15.   I notice when my mind wanders.

1	2	3	4	5	6	7
much less than before	less than before	slightly less than before	normal; no different	slightly more than before	more thsn before	much more than before

16.   I notice when my emotions or mood changes.

1	2	3	4	5	6	7
much less than before	less than before	slightly less than before	normal; no different	slightly more than before	more thsn before	much more than before

17.   My muscles feel soft and limp.

1	2	3	4	5	6	7
much less than before	less than before	slightly less than before	normal; no different	slightly more than before	more thsn before	much more than before

18.   My muscles feel different.

1	2	3	4	5	6	7
much less than before	less than before	slightly less than before	normal; no different	slightly more than before	more thsn before	much more than before

19.   I am relaxed.

1	2	3	4	5	6	7
much less than before	less than before	slightly less than before	normal; no different	slightly more than before	more thsn before	much more than before

20.   My body is heavy.

1	2	3	4	5	6	7
much less than before	less than before	slightly less than before	normal; no different	slightly more than before	more thsn before	much more than before

Appendix C
Behavioral Relaxation Scale Recording Form

SCORE SHEET

Client: _____ Setting: _____ Date: _____

Observer: _____ Activity: _____ Phase: B   TX   F

Parent/Child: _____ Session: _____ Type: PRE   POST

Breathing Baseline: _____

− unrelaxed   + relaxed   Reclined   Upright

	PRE					POST					TOTAL	
	1	2	3	4	5	1	2	3	4	5	PRE	POST
Breathing	− +	− +	− +	− +	− +	− +	− +	− +	− +	− +		
Body	− +	− +	− +	− +	− +	− +	− +	− +	− +	− +		
Head	− +	− +	− +	− +	− +	− +	− +	− +	− +	− +		
Shoulders	− +	− +	− +	− +	− +	− +	− +	− +	− +	− +		
Throat	− +	− +	− +	− +	− +	− +	− +	− +	− +	− +		
Hands	− +	− +	− +	− +	− +	− +	− +	− +	− +	− +		
Feet	− +	− +	− +	− +	− +	− +	− +	− +	− +	− +		
Eyes	− +	− +	− +	− +	− +	− +	− +	− +	− +	− +		
Mouth	− +	− +	− +	− +	− +	− +	− +	− +	− +	− +		
Quiet	− +	− +	− +	− +	− +	− +	− +	− +	− +	− +		

Self-Rating: 1 2 3 4 5 6 7   Self-Rating: 1 2 3 4 5 6 7   SCORE

Appendix D
Written Criterion Tests for Behavioral Relaxation Scale Observers

Form A

1. List the 10 items scored on the BRS.
2. Which of the following are not considered to be relaxed?
    a. Chin sunk down on chest
    b. Shoulders sloped and even
    c. Feet crossed at the ankles
    d. Eyes open and focused on the middle distance
3. What is the optimal duration for a BRS observation period?
    a. 30 minutes
    b. 30 seconds
    c. 5 minutes
    d. 5 seconds
4. If a trainee clears her throat during an observation period, this could be scored as unrelaxed . . .
    a. Mouth
    b. Quiet
    c. Breathing
    d. Throat
5. How percentage unrelaxed behavior calculated?

Form B
1. List the 10 items scored on the BRS.
2. Which of the following are scored as relaxed behavior?
    a. Eyelids closed and smooth
    b. Lips closed with corners of the mouth downturned
    c. Hands folded in lap
    d. Heels together and toes apart in a "V"
3. How long is breathing observed during each interval of the observation period?
    a. 30 seconds
    b. 30 minutes
    c. 5 seconds
    d. 5 minutes
4. If a trainee scratches his nose during an observation period, this would be scored as unrelaxed . . .
    a. Face
    b. Hands
    c. Head
    d. Body
5. How is percentage of relaxed behavior calculated?

Form C
1. List the 10 items scored on the BRS.
2. Relaxed breathing is defined as . . .
    a. The abdomen rises and falls while the shoulders remain stationary
    b. No movement of the chest, shoulders, or body
    c. Absence of interruptions such as coughing
    d. A rate slower than baseline
3. Each interval of the observation period consists of observing . . .
    a. Breathing for 20 seconds, other 9 items for 20 seconds, recording for 20 seconds
    b. 60 seconds observation for each item in succession
    c. Breathing for 30 seconds, other 9 items for 15 seconds, recording for 15 seconds
    d. All 10 items simultaneously for 60 seconds
4. If a trainee swallows during an observation period, this would be scored as unrelaxed . . .
    a. Mouth
    b. Throat
    c. Chest
    d. Body
5. What is the formula used to calculate interobserver agreement between observers?

NOTE: BRS = Behavioral Relaxation Scale.

Appendix E
Pre-Post BRT Distress Rating Form

Name: _____   Phase: Baseline   R-BRT   UBRT   FU

Instructions: When you encounter a trigger situation, or you notice that you are upset and distressed, that is a signal for you to use relaxation. Record the date and you level of distress immediate before relaxation. Relax as you have been taught for the next 15 minutes. Immediately record your distress level at the end of the relaxation session.

Subjective Unit of Distress

1	2	3	4	5	6	7	8	9	10
Very calm				Overwhelmed				agitated, can't function	

Date	Before BRT	After BRT
_____	_____	_____
_____	_____	_____
_____	_____	_____
_____	_____	_____
_____	_____	_____
_____	_____	_____
_____	_____	_____
_____	_____	_____
_____	_____	_____
_____	_____	_____

Appendix F
Contract Maintaining Behavior Change

Between _____ and _____
           (Patient),   (Healthcare Provider)

Regarding patient and provider responsibilities after the end of treatment.

Patient responsibilities

For me, _____ (patient name), to be able to maintain and further improve the results I have achieved so far, and meet my treatment goal(s) I promise to:

1. Practice relaxation at least once per day for at least 15 to 20 minutes.
2. Use mini-BRT sessions prior to encountering a known trigger situation.
3. Use mini-BRT sessions whenever my SUD rating is a 3 or greater.
4. Praise myself for taking action (using relaxation) when practicing or using relaxation in trigger situations.
5. If a setback occurs (which always happens sooner or later) during the continued practice I will:
    a. Immediately restrict it temporarily.
    b. Follow the list of instructions (#1–4 above) for these events.
    c. As a last resort, call _____ to get support and advice.
6. Mail the completed daily Pre-Post Relaxation and Distress Rating Record at the end of each week to _____ (provider's name) for the next six weeks.

Healthcare provider responsibilities

For me, _____ (name of healthcare provider), to help you maintain your success, I promise to:

1. Call you once a week for the first two weeks to provide support and encouragement.
2. Be available during telephone hours in case you need some support and advice.

Signature: _____, _____
              (Patient),   (Healthcare Provider)

Date: _____

Appendix G
Residential BRT Checklist

Name: _____ Date: _____ Time: _____

ISP Goal: ____ Joe will utilize his relaxation strategy at least 3 times per week this report period.

Antecedents: **Peer confrontation** **Being prompted to take a shower** **Being told no** **Having to wait**

            − unrelaxed   + relaxed

	−	+	−	+	−	+			TOTALS
Breathing									
Quiet	−	+	−	+	−	+			
Body	−	+	−	+	−	+			
Head	−	+	−	+	−	+			
Eyes	−	+	−	+	−	+			
Mouth	−	+	−	+	−	+			
Throat	−	+	−	+	−	+			
Shoulders	−	+	−	+	−	+			
Hands	−	+	−	+	−	+			
Feet	−	+	−	+	−	+			

Relaxation Rating: *Pre:* 1 2 3 4 5 6 7   *Post:* 1 2 3 4 5 6 7

Appendix H
Caregiver Reclined Relaxation Rating Form

Instructions:
1. Record the day of the observation.
2. Before commencing the relaxation rating _____ (patient's name) level of upset and distress using the scale below.

Anxiety/Distress Rating

1	2	3	4	5	6	7	8	9	10
Very calm				Overwhelmed, agitated,					can't function

Level of upset and distress before relaxation: _____

3. At the end of the 15-minute relaxation period, spend one minute to observe him/her relaxing. During 1-minute period, record a + next to each relaxed behavior performed correctly *during the entire 60 seconds.* Record a – next to each behavior that is unrelaxed.

Head straight and supported	+	–,
Body straight	+	–,
Eyes closed; no movement	+	–
Throat is smooth; no movement	+	–
Hands curled and on the arms of the chair	+	–,
Feet supported and in a "V" position	+	–,
Quiet; no talking or noise	+	–,
Shoulders rounded and even; supported	+	–,
Mouth open ¼ of an inch	+	–
Slow breathing from the belly	+	–

4. Rate the level of _____ upset and distress after relaxation.

Appendix I:
Reclined Relaxed BRT Acquisition Training Protocol

Reclined BRT Acquisition Training Protocol

Trainer: _____ Date: _____ O2 name: _____ IOA %: _____

Performance % correct: _____

Instructions: Record a plus (+) for each correct step; a minus (−) for each incorrect response. Record NA (not applicable) for steps that were not relevant to that trial.

Step	Trial 1	2	3	4	5	6	7	8	9	10
Label and define the behavior.										
Model relaxed and unrelaxed behavior.										
Instruct S to relax the behavior under training.										
Instruct S to notice how it feels to relax your ____.										
Instruct S to relax any previously trained behaviors.										
Observe S for 5 seconds.										
Use error correction as needed: a. Instruct S to correct behavior (one time per behavior) and wait 5 seconds for S response. b. If not correct, describe relaxed behavior and provide physical guidance. c. Give instruction to relax all behaviors, as needed.										
Observe S for 30".										
Give feedback and praise contingent on performance.										
Conduct additional training trials as needed until the behavior reaches 30" criterion (If the criterion is NOT met, go to step 3).										
New behavior added to training, when previous behavior is at criterion. (Repeat steps 2-10).										
Provides instruction at a slow and reasonable pace. Poor — Excellent	1 2 3 4 5	1 2 3 4 5	1 2 3 4 5	1 2 3 4 5	1 2 3 4 5	1 2 3 4 5	1 2 3 4 5	1 2 3 4 5	1 2 3 4 5	1 2 3 4 5
Uses a calm monotonic voice. Poor — Excellent	1 2 3 4 5	1 2 3 4 5	1 2 3 4 5	1 2 3 4 5	1 2 3 4 5	1 2 3 4 5	1 2 3 4 5	1 2 3 4 5	1 2 3 4 5	1 2 3 4 5
Training conducted for 20 minutes or all behaviors trained, instruct S to "Relax on your own for a few minutes."										
Conduct 5' BRS observation.										
At end of observation, instruct S "On the count of three slowly open your eyes."										
Praise performance; give corrective feedback.										
Ask S: "What did you...... Notice while relaxing?" Feel while relaxing?" Find most difficult to relax??"										
Provide social reinforcement and feedback based on the BRS data and self-report.										
Calculate total percentage correct for all trials	Overall %age correct:									

Name Index

A
Acosta, F. X., 127
Ajimsha, M. S., 176
Allen; R., 115
American Psychiatric Association, 115, 211
Anderson, C. A., 10
Andrasik, F., 21
Apostolova, L. G., 169
Axmom, A., 153
Arias, A. J., 130

B
Bacon, M., 96
Baer, R.A., 47, 48
Bain, P.G., 202, 218
Barkley, R. A., 131, 134
Baum, J., G., 138
Baumstark, K. E., 157
Bechtler, J., 126, 127
Beck, R., 11
Ben-Naim, S., 130
Benson, H., 23, 26, 34
Bergin, A., 212
Berkowitz, L., 9, 10
Bernstein, D. A., 19, 49, 65, 104
Biederman, J., 130
Blanchard, E. B., 19, 21, 22, 49, 67, 89, 151, 153
Blumenthal, J. A., 11
Boice, R., 63
Borkovec, T. D., 50, 172
Boyer, B.A., 96
Brennan, R., 29
Breau, L. M., 153

Brott, P., 172
Bruns, J., 21,
Budzinski, T. H., 20
Burgio, L. D., 125

C
Calamari, J. E., 115, 125
Cannon, W. B., 4, 25
Capaldi, D. M., 138
Carbray, J. ., 130
Carey, J., 172
Carr, E. G., 176
Carrington, P., 23
Castro, J., 101
Cervantes, P., 125
Chalfant, A. M., 126,127
Chan, S. W. C., 69
Chandrana, V., 197
Chapell, M. S., 173
Chen, W., 127
Chida, Y., 11
Chung, W., 176, 197
Clauw, D. J., 156
Compton, S., 172
Cone, J. D., 43
Costello, J. E., 125
Cowles, B. J., 130
Creswell, J. D., 27
Creswell, J. D., 46
Crist, D. A., 46, 228

D
Dahlhamer, J., 150
Davidson, R. J., 26
DeLisi, M., 11

Dissanayaka, N. N., 175, 176
Dollard, J., 9
Donney, V. K., 134
Ducharme, J. M., 214

E
Elble, R. J., 197
Ellgring, H., 175
Esch, T., 213,
Eufemia, R. L., 154

F
Fahn, S., 176, 198
Faraone, S. V., 130,
Fecteau, G. W., 213
Ferraro, F. R., 157
Ferster, C. B., 43
Foster, S. L., 63, 65
Fordyce, W., 49, 157
Freud, S., 6
Fried, R., 96, 97
Friedman, R. M., 138

G
Gajsak, L. R., 127
Garlovsky, J. K., 175
Gellhorn, E., 25
Giardono, L., 155
Gilliam, J. E., 138
Giggins, O. M., 21
Glancy, G., 11
Goadsby, P. J., 151
Goldstein, D., 4
Goyette, C. H., 131, 134, 138, 139
Green, E., 21
Gross, C. G., 28
Gündel, H., 173
Guercio, J. M., 216, 218
Gutkin, A. J., 42, 45

H
Hammond, K., 232
Handen, B. L., 130
Hanrahan, S., 115
Harris, R., 43, 76
Harvey, J. R., 115, 125
Haynes, S. N., 231
Headache disorders, 151
Heide, F. J., 103
Helfer, S. L., 167
Hendershot, C.S., 90
Herrnstein, R. J., 157

Hillenberg, J. B., 42, 45
Hiott, D. W., 214
Hites, L. S., 46, 228
Hobbs, C., 47
Hoelscher, T. J., 90
Hopko, D. R., 157, 173
Howes, O. D., 127
Hwang, T. J., 169

I
Iwata, B. A., 43

J
Jacobson, E., 18, 49
Jacobson, N. S., 157
Johnston, J. M., 63
Jones, L. C., 169

K
Kabat-Zinn, J., 24
Kanfer, F. H., 43, 231
Kaushik, R., 96, 97
Kehoe, E. J., 157
Kennedy, S., 153
Kessler, R. C., 150, 172
Kiesel, K. B., 43, 118, 125
Knapp, M. L., 32
Kosek, E., 156, 157
Krmpotich, J. D., 91

L
LaChapelle, D. L., 153
Lau, M. A., 48
Lehrer, P. M., 26, 46,
Lettow, L., 47
Ley, R., 97
Liberman, R. P., 115
Linden, W., 21
Lindsay, W. R., 11, 120, 121, 122, 125, 140
Lister, K. E., 231
Lodge, D. J., 127
Louis, E. D., 175, 197, 198
Luiselli, J. K., 46, 67, 115, 125
Lundervold, D. A., 47, 58, 76, 86, 107, 125, 157, 169, 172, 175, 176, 178, 187, 198, 200, 228, 229, 231

M
Main, C., 76
Marlott, G. A., 90
Martinez-Raga, J., 130
Mash, E. J., 130

Marx, R. D., 90
Masserman, J., 6
Mattick, R. P., 198
Matthews, A. M., 48
May, M. A., 153
McCracken, L. M., 157
McGimpsey, B. A., 115, 116
McGuire, B.E., 153
McLaughlin, K., 11
McManus, S., 153
McPhali, C. H., 115
Michultka, D., 153
Morley, S., 232
Mostofsky, E., 11
Mruzek, D. W., 90
Murphy, K. R., 130
Musacchio, T., 175
Myin-Germeys, I., 115

N
National Institute of Neurological and Communication Disorders, 211
Newman, M. G., 103
Noe, S. R., 127, 130
Norton, M., 48, 66, 68,69
Novaco, R. W., 11, 139

O
Ortega, D. F., 115
O'Neill, R. E., 231
O'Sullivan, S. S., 175
Overall, J. E., 128

P
Pachana, N. A., 2
Paclawski, T. R., 117, 120
Pavlov, I., 6
Peper, E., 96, 97
Perepletchikova, F., 42, 45
Pharr, O. M., 127
Phillips, L. J., 127
Poppen, R., 7, 26, 27, 35, 68, 69, 91, 166, 227, 231
Potvin, O., 169

Q
Qualls, P. J., 48

R
Rashid, Z. M., 172
Raymer, R. H., 131
Reaven, J., 126, 127
Reinking, R. H., 48, 89

Reiss, S., 115,
Rickard, H. C., 127, 129,
Roemer, L., 47
Rosenblatt, A., 213, 214
Rutten, S., 176

S
Schilling, D. J., 19, 46, 48, 65, 66, 67, 68, 69, 72, 139
Scheufele, P. M., 69, 226
Schlesinger, I., 176, 71
Schneier, F. R., 175, 198
Schultz, J. H., 22
Schwarz, G. E., 5
Segool, N. K., 172
Selye, H., 5
Sheikh, J. I., 2
Simonoff, E., 125
Singh, N. N., 115, 120
Skinner, B. F., 29, 31, 33, 35, 42, 43, 44, 48, 76, 102
Smith, J. C., 46, 47, 228
Spielberger, C. D., 128, 173
Stahl, J. E., 11
Storch, E. A., 126, 127
Sturmey, P., 115
Sukhodolsky, D. G., 126, 127
Sur, J., 69
Szabo, S., 5

T
Tafrate, R. C., 11
Tang, W. K., 169
Tarlow, K. R., 181, 232
Tarnowski, K. J., 178, 182
Tatum, T., 173, 187
Taylor, D. N., 48
Taylor, J. L., 11, 115, 120
Taylor, S. L., 214
Thanvi, B., 178
Thyer, B. A., 176
Tourette Association of America, 211
Travis, F., 27
Turk, D. C., 157

U
Ulrich, R., 10

V
Vancampfort, D., 127
van Steensel, F. J. A., 125
van Winkel, R., 127

von der Embse, N., 172
Vrijens, D., 169

W
Walitt, B., 156
Walker, H. M., 172
Walkup, A., 65
Wallace, R. K., 26
Walsh, M., 153
Wenzel, T., 175
Wheeler, J. J., 42, 45
White, K. P., 156
White, S. W., 125
Wilder, D. A., 42, 45
Williams, J., 11
Williams, J. M. G., 24
Whitaker, S., 115, 120
Wittrock, D. A., 67, 68, 228
Wolpe, J., 2, 6, 7, 18, 25, 46, 49, 166, 167
Wu, J., 29
Yesavage, J. A., 176
Yeaton, W. H., 42, 45
Yody, B. B., 214
Zahara, D. J., 214
Zaja, R. H., 3
Zettle, R., 39, 44, 76, 89
Zollman, F. S., 214

Subject Index

A

Activities of daily living (ADL): 140, 200, 201, 204, 216, 220, 260

Aggression/aggressive behavior: 3, 4, 9–13, 31, 116, 120, 121, 125, 130, 138, 139, 141, 142 154, 233, 260

Anger: 4, 6, 9–13,26, 30, 32, 33, 69, 115, 116, 120, 138, 139, 142, 146, 156, 212

   clinical diagnosis: Intermittent Explosive Disorder (IED) 10, 11, 13, 254, 260

Anxiety: 1, 4, 5–7, 17, 18, 26, 29–33, 36, 47, 49, 75, 76, 89, 116, 140, 143, 189–193

   assessment:

      Abbreviated Test Anxiety Scale (ATAS) 173, 174

      Clinical Anxiety Scale (CAS), 176, 182, 184, 185, 193

      Geriatric Anxiety Inventory (GAI) 2, 12, 263

      Pain Anxiety Symptom Score (PASS) 157–165

      State Trait Anxiety Inventory (STAI) 69, 72, 144, 173,191,

      basic research: 6,7

   clinical diagnosis: Generalized Anxiety, 8, 47, 103, 111, 191

   Panic, 7, 8, 32,89, 111, 166, 230,

   Phobia, 7, 8, 18, 31, 157, 166, 167, 169, 171, 172, 190–193, 198

   Post Traumatic Stress Disorder, 7

   comorbid: 125, 126

   occurrence in: Autism Spectrum Disorder (ASD), 125–127

      Educational settings, 172–175

      Essential Tremor (ET), 198, 220

      Intellectual Disability (ID), 116, 121–124

      Movement disorder, 175–187

      Pain disorder, 157–166

      Schizophrenic Spectrum Disorder (SDS), 127–130

      Traumatic Brain Injury (TBI), 214, 222

   relaxation-induced anxiety (RIA), 100, 103, 111

Any anxiety disorder, 7

Attention deficit hyperactivity disorder (ADHD): 115, 130, 131–134, 136–138, 145, 212

Autism/Autism Spectrum Disorder (ASD): 3, 43, 70, 111, 115, 125, 143, 230, 233

Autogenic training/autogenic phrases: 22, 35, 38, 47, 192, 227, 230

Autonomic nervous system: 4, 21, 25, 32, 37, 157, 197

   parasympathetic arousal: 25

   sympathetic arousal: 21, 25, 26, 101

Avoidance: 2, 6, 8, 31, 43, 89, 157, 158, 165, 214

B

Behavior categories

   covert: 28, 29, 49, 172

   overt: 10, 28, 29, 121, 172, 220

   motor: 29, 30, 33, 34, 35, 37, 47–49, 676, 70–72, 87, 103, 115, 121, 123, 140, 151, 157, 166, 175–178, 191, 192, 211, 213–215, 218, 226–230

   observational: 33–35, 37, 61, 64, 68, 73, 85, 87, 88, 102, 103, 109, 123, 129, 140. 166, 214, 226–230

verbal: 35–39, 44, 48, 49, 57, 68, 69, 78, 79, 85, 96, 102–106, 109, 117, 121–125, 129, 134, 140, 150, 153, 154, 157, 166, 211, 218 226–230
visceral: 37, 48, 68, 70, 87, 95, 96, 103, 104, 126, 140, 150, 151, 166, 226–230
Behavioral assessment: 15, 40, 42, 43, 71–76, 89, 113, 148, 179, 195, 224, 228, 233
Behavioral Relaxation Scale (BRS)
 behavior definitions: 50–57
 history: 49,50
 modifications: 69, 118, 121
 observation procedure: 61–63, 77–79, 85–88 96, 101, 135, 156, 170, 179, 213
 observer training: 63–65
 performance criteria: 83, 84, 86, 87, 99, 105, 106, 117, 118, 128, 131,132, 137, 138, 154, 170, 189, 198, 199, 201, 202, 205, 206, 215 209, 229, 234
 reliability: 64 73, 117, 128, 131, 135, 202, 228
 scoring: 60–63, 88, 95, 99
 validity: 65, 67–70, 72, 228
Behavioral Relaxation Training (BRT)
 acquisition: 20, 78–84, 90, 94, 105–109, 111, 128, 138, 140, 142, 154, 173
 home practice: 89, 102, 110, 126, 128, 129, 134, 213
 maintenance: 88. 90, 102, 194, 106, 110, 125, 128, 138, 140, 141, 160, 214
 problems: 100–104
 proficiency: 63, 64, 75, 77, 78, 84–87, 96, 99, 106, 109, 117, 126, 131, 132, 135, 138, 154 170, 173, 184, 215, 228, 230
 rationale: 35, 36, 60, 76–78, 102, 104, 110, 151, 152, 167, 179, 227
 setting: 20, 35, 59, 62, 63, 77, 90, 91, 103, 104 107,119, 122, 141, 170, 229
 training student trainers: 107–110
 training parent trainers: 132–138
Biofeedback: 33, 35,
 electromyographic (EMG): 20, 21, 35, 65–68 72, 103, 111, 127, 131, 140, 144, 155, 188, 192, 199–201, 204–212, 216–222, 227, 229–233
 thermal (TEMP): 21, 22, 35, 37, 38, 73, 151, 152, 230
Brain:
 injury: 197, 214, 217–219, 221, 222, 230
 stimulation: 176
 tumor: 161
Breathing: 3, 8, 28, 29. 32–35, 68, 103, 111, 120
 Focused: 75, 83, 91, 95–100

 in Autogenic Training: 22
 in BRT: 19, 57–63, 76, 79, 83–87, 95, 102, 117, 118, 121, 129, 152, 153, 162, 179. 213
 in Clinical Standardized Meditation: 24
 in Mindfulness-Based Stress Reduction: 24
 in Relaxation Response: 23

C
Choreiform movement: 213, 214
Conners Teacher Rating Scale/Questionnaire: 131, 133, 134, 137–139, 145
Contracting: 90, 106, 111, 112, 213
Coping: 2, 4, 11, 26, 43, 126, 129, 130, 176, 179–181, 184, 187, 207

D
Depression: 11, 130, 156–158, 160, 162, 166, 175–177, 179, 182, 184–186, 189–191, 193, 203
 Geriatric Depression Scale (GDS): 2, 12, 157, 161, 176, 182, 184, 186, 189, 193
Developmental disability: 11, 13, 70, 71, 115, 118, 139, 141–143, 188, 193
Diagnostic and Statistical Manual (DSM): 7, 10, 12, 127, 141, 221
Differential reinforcement: 40, 121, 124
Differential relaxation: 18, 20, 95
Disruptive behavior: 106, 121, 125, 130, 138–140, 179, 212

E
Electrodermal response (EDR): 32, 128
Emotional arousal/ behavior/distress/ reaction: 8, 11, 12, 24, 25–27, 29, 30, 36, 38, 43, 115, 118, 121, 141, 150, 157, 175, 182, 190, 197, 212–214
Emotional Disturbance (ED): 138, 142, 239
Escape: 5, 8, 29, 31, 33, 43, 157, 165, 214

F
Fibromyalgia: 110, 156–165, 189, 230
Fight-or-flight response: 4, 5, 8, 12, 21, 23, 25, 29
Functional analysis: 3, 42, 43,71, 226
Functional assessment: 3, 12, 15, 43, 74, 113, 195, 224, 233

H
Headache: 11, 18, 19, 26, 37, 38, 44, 49, 73, 76, 97, 105, 110, 130, 151, 188, 229
 Headache Index: 152, 153
 migraine: 5, 20. 96, 151–153, 157, 162
 mixed: 153, 154
 tension: 5, 21, 22, 37, 70, 72, 75, 110, 144, 151, 154, 155, 230

Home practice: 19, 20, 22, 24, 35, 89, 100, 102, 110, 117, 126, 128, 129, 134, 213
Huntington's Disease: 213, 214, 221
Hyperactivity Index: 131, 133, 134, 138
Hypertension: 5, 18, 21, 24–26, 38, 49, 67, 73, 111, 229, 230, 233
Hyperventilation: 71, 98, 101, 111, 118, 119, 125, 142
Hypnogogic jerk: 101

I

Imagery: 27, 28, 33, 75, 98, 103, 138, 151, 179–181, 192, 230
Informed consent: 158, 231
Instruction: 11, 14, 19–21, 23, 29–31, 33, 35, 36, 39, 40, 48, 59, 60, 65, 66, 76, 79, 83, 85, 87 96, 102, 105, 107, 112, 116, 117, 121, 124, 140 147, 153, 158, 164, 167, 173, 182, 187, 212, 219, 223, 234
  self-instruction: 28, 124, 125, 138, 140, 153, 156
Intermittent Explosive Disorder DSM-5 312.34 11
Interobserver agreement: 74, 126, 147, 158, 194, 223
Intellectual Disability (ID): 5, 11, 13, 43, 69, 115–118, 121–125, 127, 141–143, 153, 188, 230, 233
Interval observation: 61, 85, 109

M

Maintenance: 29, 70, 88. 90. 102, 104, 106, 110 113, 117, 125, 128, 138, 141, 148, 160, 214
Medication: 1, 2, 5, 11, 43, 45, 107, 116, 118, 127, 130, 131, 134, 145, 150, 154–158, 160, 162, 165, 166, 170, 176, 177, 182, 184, 204, 212, 213
Meditation: 22–24, 27, 34, 35, 38, 47, 72, 76, 96 103, 127, 227
Mindfulness: 24, 38, 47, 48, 72, 142, 232
Mini-relaxation: 35, 75, 91, 95, 100, 107, 110, 152, 156,
Motivational interview: 44, 76
Motivating operations: 14, 44, 141, 194, 223

O

Operant: 6, 10, 16, 96, 112, 114, 147, 149, 157, 194, 196, 223, 225

P

Pain: 75, 76, 97, 110, 130, 150, 151–153
  back: 5, 162, 189, 229, 230
  chronic: 73, 110, 150, 153, 157, 158, 162, 187–189, 230
  neurofacial: 155, 188
Parkinson's disease: 5, 176–178, 180, 181, 191–193, 198, 200, 221
Placebo: 44, 48, 65–67, 69, 227
Pliance/ply: 35, 44, 70, 89, 90, 106, 111, 212
Progressive (Muscle) Relaxation (PMR): 17, 18, 21, 24, 27, 37, 38, 67, 71, 73, 103, 111, 120, 142, 144, 151, 176, 229, 232
Punishment: 10, 16, 34, 89

R

Reactivity: 58, 59
Reciprocal inhibition: 12, 25, 37, 71, 76, 110, 190
Reinforcement/reinforcer/reinforcing consequences: 6, 9, 10, 14, 16, 29, 31, 34, 36, 39, 40, 43–45, 71, 74, 76, 77, 85, 86, 90, 102, 105–107, 110, 112, 114, 117, 121, 124, 128–130, 132, 140, 141, 147, 149, 157, 158, 166, 176, 177, 190, 194, 213, 223, 225, 231
Relaxation Inventory: 46, 47, 71, 232
Relaxation Response (RR): 13, 23, 26, 27, 38,
Replacement behavior: 11, 27, 43, 89, 23
Respondent conditioning: 6–8, 10, 16, 32,149, 157, 196
Response class: 16, 26, 34, 41, 68, 74, 114, 149, 157, 196, 225, 226, 228
Rules/rule-governed behavior: 16, 35, 36, 39, 40, 44, 71, 76, 89, 110, 112, 147, 150, 227

S

Self-report: 9, 30–32, 36, 42, 45–49, 65, 69–72, 78, 89, 103, 116, 117, 120, 127–129, 131, 152, 160, 162, 168, 173, 174, 187, 204, 215, 216, 220, 227–232
Single-subject research: 158, 181, 203, 213, 230, 231, 232
States of Arousal and Relaxation (STAR): 47, 72, 233
Stress: 1, 2–5, 7, 8, 11–13, 17, 23–27, 36, 38, 43, 44, 65, 66, 69, 71, 73, 75, 76, 89, 90, 96, 101, 110, 115, 116, 127, 130, 142, 144, 145, 150–153, 155–157, 175, 176, 182, 184, 187, 197, 198, 212, 213, 221, 230, 232, 233
Subjective Units of Distress Scale (SUDS) 2, 46, 167, 170–174, 177–186, 198
Systematic Desensitization: 18, 72, 166–169, 190

T

Theories of relaxation: 24
  Autonomic (unitary): 25

Brain-State: 27
Cognitive-Somatic (dualistic): 26
Four-Modality Response System: 27
Muscular: 25
Tokens: 105, 106, 112, 126, 131, 132, 135, 147
Tourette Syndrome: 211, 221,
Tremor: 157, 175, 181, 182, 184, 191, 192, 197–211, 216–222, 233

U

Upright BRS (UBRS): 69, 91, 156, 159, 162, 164, 180, 182–185, 199, 202, 205–208, 229

Upright BRT (UBRT): 2, 19, 75, 89, 91–95, 100, 110, 111, 156, 158–160, 162–165, 170, 172–175, 177–185, 187, 191, 198, 199, 201–206, 209–211

V

Values clarification: 43, 76
Values for living: 2, 76, 90, 102

Behavioral Relaxation Training: Clinical Applications with Diverse Populations, Third Edition is a welcome update to a valuable clinical resource. It provides a rigorous behavioral conceptual and data-based methodological framework in a highly user-friendly manner, readily lending itself to practical application of the effective procedures to socially relevant behaviors. This latest edition expands the client populations and behavior challenges that are addressed, accompanied with supportive data.

The authors candidly note the varying strength of the supporting data for various specific applications of BRT and set the occasion for continuing research with the procedures. A really nice touch is the provision for each chapter of items from the Behavior Analyst Certification Board Task List (5th edition) that correspond to the concepts and procedures addressed in it. Further, linking the rationale and procedures for BRT to basic behavioral research as well as to work done in non-behavior analytic framework adds to this book's value. As a person who has been using BRT in my clinical work for years, I welcome this expanded presentation of work in the area.

— Dr. Gordon Bourland, Trinity Behavioral Services, Fort Worth, TX

In my career, I have found a handful of resources that I believe belong close at hand to every clinician, applied researcher, and student of human service fields. *Behavioral Relaxation Training: Clinical Applications with Diverse Populations, Third Edition* is one of them. I have always been very impressed with the simple elegance of BRT and its adaptability to the gamut of applications so well covered in this volume.

The reader is immediately exposed to a view of the range of applicability of BRT. Each chapter subsequently exposes the reader to a review of the basic components of BRT, its research and clinical history, means for measuring relaxation, rules for relaxation, and of considerable importance, the role of the trainer. Chapters also have relevant supplements providing additional details of assessments and measures and other relevant information such as Behavior Analyst certification.

The entire book is like BRT itself, simply elegant. It is easy to read, magnificently thorough without in any way being cumbersome, and at the same time, concise. It will be remarkably useful for clinicians and researchers to use it with a singular problem of focus, or with the panoply of disorders covered. It is a gift to clinicians and researchers.

— Dr. John R. Lutzker, Professor Emeritus, Georgia State University

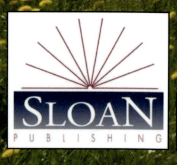

Sloan Publishing
220 Maple Road
Cornwall on Hudson, NY 12520